Mental health care delivery: innovations, impediments and
implementation

Mental health care delivery: innovations, impediments and implementation

Edited by

ISAAC M. MARKS

Institute of Psychiatry, University of London and Bethlem–Maudsley Hospital, London, SE5 8AF, UK

ROBERT A. SCOTT

Center for Advanced Study in the Behavioral Sciences, Stanford, CA94305, USA

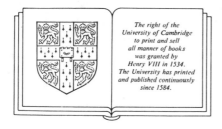

The right of the
University of Cambridge
to print and sell
all manner of books
was granted by
Henry VIII in 1534.
The University has printed
and published continuously
since 1584.

CAMBRIDGE UNIVERSITY PRESS

Cambridge

New York   Port Chester

Melbourne   Sydney

Published by the Press Syndicate of the University of Cambridge
The Pitt Building, Trumpington Street, Cambridge CB2 1RP
40 West 20th Street, New York NY 10011, USA
10 Stamford Road, Oakleigh, Melbourne 3166, Australia

First published 1990

Printed in Great Britain at the University Press, Cambridge

British Library cataloguing in publication data
Mental health care delivery: innovations, impediments and implementation.
1. Mentally ill persons. Care
I. Marks, Isaac M. (Isaac Meyer), 1935–   II. Scott, Robert
362.2'0425

Library of Congress cataloguing in publication data
Mental health care delivery: innovations, impediments and
implementation / edited by Isaac Marks, Robert Scott.
    p.   cm.
ISBN 0 521 38494 X
1. Mental health services—Administration.   2. Mental health
services.   I. Marks, Isaac Meyer.   II. Scott, Robert A., 1935–
[DNLM: 1. Mental Health Services—organization & administration.
2. Mental Health Services—trends.   WM 30 M5447]
RA790.5.M419   1990
362.2'068—dc20
DNLM/DLC
for Library of Congress   89-25178 CIP

ISBN 0 521 38494 X

Contents

Foreword

Norman Sartorius

There is a paradox in modern management: instead of searching for what has worked well and continues to work well so as to preserve it and be proud of it, managers are invited to seek innovations, to laud innovators, to try out new ways of doing things.

Trying out new ways of doing things is justified and wise if there are problems for which none of the known solutions seems adequate. In other instances, introducing an innovation is an unjustified and unnecessary risk which may harm the service, decrease its capacity and waste resources.

The crucial question for a decision about innovation is then what should be considered an adequate solution. Placing elderly demented patients in draughty hospital corridors where they caught pneumonia which ended their life was considered a sensible solution a few decades ago; today this is not so but there are undoubtedly services which we consider adequate now but which will be rejected in the future as obsolete, inhumane or inappropriate.

How can we know whether our judgment that a solution is adequate, is correct? Minimal standards of care, technological possibilities, ethical requirements, perception of human rights all change in time and cannot inform us when to stop 'improving' because any further tinkering may detract from the value of a set of interventions. Relying on empirical evidence is also usually not possible: proposals for true innovations do not come with a thick file of results showing how well they worked in the setting in which they are to be applied.

The problem of when to try to do better is obviously not specific to psychiatric services, medicine or social services: it is a problem relevant to all activities of governments, to our own lives and decisions, and to decisions of the community in which we happen to live. It can never be resolved but risks arising — whatever choice we decide to take — can be significantly reduced if we listen to the experience of others who have tried an innovation similar to the one contemplated; if we introduce innovations gradually, learning from the results of their application in parts of the system before extending them to other parts; if we decide and clearly state what the main criteria for 'better' in our setting are; and if we monitor progress towards improvement, retaining a constant readiness to reject an innovation as soon as the results of its application do not satisfy a reasonable mix of requirements of patients, their families and communities.

This book brings together experience in the use of innovations, documented as well as possible, from different institutions and settings. It also summarizes issues and points that arose in the in-depth debate of an interdisciplinary group which examined these presentations. It can thus be seen as a list of inspiring examples, as a catalogue of possibilities and an assembly of warnings to those who are in charge of mental health services, who teach about them or who study their functioning. In this way it is an important step in the search for better, more humane and more efficient services.

Mental health care is a vast subject, and it was clearly necessary to choose a few topics of particular importance. Thus among types of mental health services mainly three have been focussed on: community care for those with chronic psychosis, the mental health components of primary care, and emergency services. Numerous other types of services could have been added — from services for those with problems related to substance abuse to services provided to people about to die. The decision to include only the three listed can be justified by the significant public health and humanitarian issues arising in the care for the chronically ill in the community; by the pervasiveness of primary health care which still does not seem to be ready to include mental health components in its functioning to an extent commensurate with the size and nature of problems with which it has to deal; and by the current controversy about emergency services in the northern hemisphere countries.

Similarly, a choice had to be made among the many possible ways of classifying impediments to innovation, and describing their relative importance. They were finally divided into socio-political, administrative, economic and professional groups which allowed the reduction of the unavoidable overlap of these groups. Lack of time and space, however, meant that certain impediments had to be left out — for example the lack of feedback of needs of service delivery into undergraduate medical curricula.

Finally, a word of praise about the editors of this book. They have done much work, both administrative and technical, to produce an outstanding volume. Their attitude and strategy in doing this deserve a special mention. From the beginning of the process of producing this volume till its appearance they have sought advice from knowledgeable individuals, consulted their future authors, adjusting the course of their work so as to produce a book of value which expresses the considered views of a group of experts of different backgrounds, disciplines, nationalities and connections. In this they have succeeded admirably.

Norman Sartorius, MD, MA, PhD, DPM, FRCPsych
Director, Division of Mental Health, World Health Organization, Geneva

Acknowledgements

We gratefully acknowledge the Henry J. Kaiser Foundation and the Center/FFRP Fund for providing generous support to convene the conference out of which this volume developed. We also thank the Center for Advanced Study in the Behavioral Sciences, Stanford, for making its facility available for the meeting. Finally, we thank the Center staff for their help and acknowledge Nancy Pinkerton for her exceptionally able administrative assistance in helping us to organize the venture and complete the final manuscript.

Isaac M. Marks, London
Robert A. Scott, Stanford
November 1989

Editors

Isaac M MARKS, MD, FRCPsych, Professor of Experimental Psychopathology and Consultant Psychiatrist, Institute of Psychiatry, University of London and Bethlem–Maudsley Hospital, London SE5 8AF, UK

Robert A SCOTT PhD, Deputy Director, Center for Advanced Study in the Behavioral Sciences, Stanford, CA94305, USA

Contributors

John CARRIER PhD, London School of Economics, Houghton Street, London WC2, UK

John E COOPER MD, FRCPsych, Professor of Psychiatry, University of Nottingham, Mapperley Hospital, Porchester Road, Nottingham, UK

Karyn C GILL, 10 Mitchell Lane, Woodbridge, CT 06525, USA

John HOULT MB BS DPM FRANZCP, Community Health Services, 184 Glebe Point Rd, Glebe, NSW 2037, Australia

Wayne KATON MD, Associate Professor, Chief, Consultation/Liaison Service, Department of Psychiatry and Behavioral Sciences, University of Washington Medical School, Seattle, WA 98195, USA

Heinz KATSCHNIG MD, Professor, Psychiatric Clinic, University of Vienna, Währinger Gürtel 18–20, A — 1090, Vienna, Austria

Gerald L KLERMAN MD, Formerly Administrator of US Alcohol, Drug Abuse and Mental Health Administration (ADAMHA); now Professor of Psychiatry and Associate Chairman for Research, Department of Psychiatry, New York Hospital-Cornell University Medical Center, 21 Bloomingdale Road, White Plains, NY 10605, USA

Martin KNAPP PhD, Professor, Personal and Social Services Research Unit, Cornwallis Building, University of Kent at Canterbury, Canterbury, Kent CT2 7NF, UK

Terese KONIECZNA, PhD, Ludwig Boltzmann Institute for Social Psychiatry, Spitalgasse 11, A-1090 Vienna, Austria

Julian LEFF MD, FRCPsych, Professor and Director of Medical Research Council Social Psychiatry Unit, Institute of Psychiatry, University of

London, Consultant Psychiatrist, Bethlem–Maudsley Hospital, London SE5 8AF, UK

Theodore R MARMOR PhD, Professor of Public Management and Political Science, Yale School of Organization and Management, 111 Prospect Street, New Haven, CT 06520, USA

Herbert PARDES MD, President, American Psychiatric Association, Formerly Director, US National Institute of Mental Health; now Professor, College of Physicians and Surgeons, Columbia University, 722 West 168th Street, New York, NY 10032, USA

Eugene S PAYKEL MA, MD, FRCP, FRCPsych, Professor of Psychiatry, University of Cambridge, Addenbrooke's Hospital, Hills Road, Cambridge CB2 2QQ, UK

Jeffrey RUBIN PhD, Associate Professor, Dept of Economics, and Core Faculty Member, Institute for Health, Health Care Policy and Aging Research, Rutgers, State University of New Jersey, New Brunswick, NJ 08903, USA

Norman SARTORIUS MD, MA, PhD, DPM, FRCPsych, Director, Division of Mental Health, World Health Organization, Geneva, Switzerland

Steven P SEGAL PhD, Professor and Director, Mental Health and Social Welfare Research Group, University of California at Berkeley, and Institute for Scientific Analysis, California 94720, USA

Mary Ann TEST PhD, Professor, Department of Social Work, University of Wisconsin, Madison, WI 53 706, USA

Sir Henry YELLOWLEES KCB, FRCP, FRCS, FFCM, Formerly Chief Medical Officer, UK Department of Health and Social Security, 43 Sandwich House, Sandwich Street, London WC1H 9PR, UK

1

Introduction

Isaac M. Marks and Robert A. Scott

Changes in paradigms for mental health care delivery are accelerating. They have been gathering momentum over the last few years and are likely to culminate in the 1990s in major shifts in many countries. The 1989 White Paper on the Health Service in the United Kingdom and the advent of a fresh Administration in the United States are giving this process further impetus. In turbulent times it can be hard to stand back and track long-term trends, though the new science of chaos teaches us that even in a maelstrom we may be able to find ordered patterns emerging. This volume is dedicated to that aim, to get a clearer view by examining a few general principles that seem to operate across the various systems of mental health care delivery in different Western countries. The book outlines some promising innovations of recent years, goes on to analyse some of the main impediments to their implementation into health care systems, and finally describes some prospects for overcoming these obstacles.

To obtain the broad scope necessary to achieve such a task, this volume is multidisciplinary. It is written by eminent psychiatrists, psychologists, social scientists, social workers, economists, and administrators who have been involved in the political process that is so crucial in shaping the final service product. Contributors are prominent experts in mental health services who have worked in the United States and the United Kingdom, continental Europe, Australia, and in the World Health Organization. The similar and contrasting experiences across different countries are illuminating. Many of the contributors met at a stimulating conference ('Innovations in Mental Health Care Delivery: Impediments and Implementation' sponsored by the Kaiser Family Foundation and the Center/FFRP Fund and held at the Center for Advanced Study in the Behavioral Sciences in

Stanford, California). Their chapters are an up-to-date account of many important issues in mental health care delivery today. They hope to interest all mental health care professionals and administrators who are trying to arrange a better deal for sufferers in a constraining world.

Rationale

Provision of effective, reasonable-cost mental health services to all sectors of the population is one of the most pressing problems facing planners and administrators of mental health services in advanced industrial societies. Everywhere, funding for human services is stringent, and strong efforts are being mounted to cap and eventually further reduce human services costs. As a result, mental health along with other human services is under growing pressure to economize. At the same time, there is pressure to improve services for categories of mental patients, such as the chronically and severely disabled, the elderly, children and minorities, which in the past have been greatly underserved. The confluence of these forces has placed a premium on the development of types of programs and forms of clinical management and treatment for mental patients, including especially underserved groups, that are less costly yet effective clinically.

In this regard, programs that are based in the community are of special interest. There are several reasons why this is so. Fiscal issues are primary. It is generally acknowledged that hospital-based programs of care are extremely costly[1] while there is every reason to expect that programs which manage and treat mental disorders in the community, where properly organized and implemented, will, in the long run, be less expensive. In addition, disillusionment remains with the old-time mental asylum as an appropriate setting for treating mental illness. The sentiment persists that removing individuals from the community and sequestering them in large, drab, often overcrowded hospital settings may cause long-term harm greater than the potential short-term good from their treatment there. Finally, it is recognized that the stigma of becoming known as a mental patient can be better mitigated by dealing with mental disorders in the community than in institutional settings. For all these reasons, there has been a strong disposition to care for mental disorder outside hospitals, resorting to admission only when this becomes absolutely necessary.

In the past few decades significant initiatives to provide psychiatric care within the community have occurred. Indeed, by now an impressive body of research has shown that such innovations in mental health care can be effective. Research on community programs indicates that they have dramatically decreased hospitalization, reduced chronicity, and increased the rate of return to a reasonably normal social life. From studies of emergency mental health services, community care programs, and mental health manpower experiments, the evidence mounts that communities which mobilize resources quickly when psychiatric crises arise can sharply reduce admission even for people who are severely ill and socially marginal; that it is feasible and effective to provide psychiatric care in primary care settings; that community care of the mentally ill, including the severely disabled, can be effective; and that the costs of training personnel to deliver many mental health services can be greatly curtailed by extending the clinical role of nurses and other personnel without the MD or PhD. Encouraging features of these demonstration studies are that costs are generally no higher than for existing methods of care, and in some cases a good deal lower; and that long-term savings accrue to the community from lower subsequent use of resources by formerly distressed people who have improved.

This point is often overlooked in the furor surrounding deinstitutionalization of the mentally ill that currently abounds. There is little question that deinstitutionalization has largely failed in the United States. Evidence for it is everywhere: in the problems of the homeless, in the development of psychiatric ghettoes in the cities, in high death rates among discharged mental patients due to neglect and lack of supervision, and so on. Yet, in the rush to correct the failings of this policy, which in the United States presently entails a powerful counterpressure to reinstitutionalize such persons, sight has been lost of the fact that deinstitutionalization of the mentally ill and community care of the mentally ill are not synonymous. Deinstitutionalization entails little more than emptying out mental hospitals by discharging patients back to the community with little regard for what happens to them once they get there. Community care for the mentally ill entails psychiatric and social programs of care, treatment and supervision of mental patients that are ongoing and comprehensive in character. It is programs of this kind we have in mind when we assert that community treatment of the mentally ill has proven successful. Indeed, one purpose of the conference and this volume was to call attention to this fact about community care of the mentally ill.

Evaluation research on these programs suggests there is good reason to hope that mental health services can be significantly improved, even with constrained resources. A great frustration is that no country in Western Europe or North America has succeeded in implementing on a large scale the organizational and clinical innovations that the research evidence suggests will work. In each nation, services are best for the dominant groups and worst for the poor. In every country there are rigidities and a prodigal waste of resources which, if redirected within a more flexible framework, could lead to the provision of effective services to all segments of society.

The papers in this volume try to shed light on why this is so. In particular, they describe several major innovations in community care for the mentally ill; analyse the principal obstacles to implementing them system-wide in the United States and the United Kingdom; and identify strategies, attempted or contemplated, for overcoming these barriers.

The book is divided into three sections. Part I describes a number of innovations in community care of persons with psychiatric illness that have been developed during the past two to three decades. They include: (a) programs for psychotic patients (Chapters 2–4); (b) primary care-based psychiatric services for non-psychotic problems (Chapters 5–6); and (c) emergency services in community settings (Chapters 7–8).

Part II analyses some impediments to implementing the sorts of innovative programs that are discussed in Part I. Four major impediments to their implementation on a system-wide basis are considered. They are: (s) sociopolitical influences on mental health care policy in the United Kingdom and Continental Europe (Chapters 9–11); (b) administrative barriers to implementing community care programs (Chapters 12–14); and, finally, (c) economic and professional barriers to disseminating such innovations (Chapters 15–17).

Part III integrates the book, provides an overview, and details some issues concerning the system-wide implementation of innovation.

To achieve reasonable depth of coverage and to avoid becoming too diffuse, this book concentrated on services for adults in Western rather than in developing countries. It inevitably had to omit the elderly, children, mental handicap, organic problems, substance abuse, and forensic and liaison psychiatry. Also outside the scope of this volume are advances in medication and in family therapy, and the advent of effective behavioural treatment for phobic/panic, obsessive–compulsive, habit and sexual disorders.

The innovations described in this volume mainly concern mental health care delivery for adults with psychotic and nonpsychotic disorders. These terms are used more in an administrative than in a clinical sense. Psychotic disorder refers mainly to schizophrenia and severe affective disorders. Traditionally, they have usually been treated as inpatients but, now they are frequently treated outside hospital. 'Nonpsychotic disorders' refers to less severe affective disorders, as well as anxiety and personality disorders. They cause handicap which in the past often went unrecognized, and when recognized were dealt with in the community, usually in a primary care setting. This division between psychotic and nonpsychotic disorders is, of course, arbitrary but reminds us that the two groups have had rather different approaches to site and methods of treatment.

With psychoses the chief innovation is the trend to manage sufferers in the community rather than in hospital. With nonpsychotic disorders, the innovation is their better recognition in the community; sufferers rarely attend mental hospitals. Only recently has it been realized that they form a large part of the clientele asking for help in primary care, psychiatric and medical outpatients, and emergency units, and consume much of the health care budget in most countries. Even today it is not yet widely realized that the vague terms 'minor psychiatric disorder' and 'neurotic disorder' often used to describe such sufferers conceals the major and chronic disability that their problem causes them and their families (Weissman, 1989). This disability can be greatly reduced by newer treatments such as behavioural psychotherapy which have appeared in the last few years (Marks, 1986, 1987), advances which are outside the main scope of this volume. Instead, we will pass on to an innovative theme that will recur throughout the book, that of community care for psychotic disorders.

Note

1. In 1983 it cost \$46,730 to maintain one patient in a mental hospital in the USA for one year (Green, 1986, pp. 23 and 28).

References

Greene, S., Witkin, M. J., Atay, J., Fell, A. & Manderscheid, R. W. (1986). State and County Mental Hospitals, United States, 1982–83, 1983–84, with Trend Analysis for 1977–74 to 1983–84. *Mental Health Statistical Note* Number 176, Rockville, Maryland, NIMH.

Marks, I. M. (1986). *Behavioural Psychotherapy: Maudsley Pocketbook of Clinical Management.* Butterworths, London.

Marks, I. M. (1987). *Fears, Phobias and Rituals.* Oxford University Press, NY.

Weissmann, M. M. (1989).Paper to Regional Conference on Biological Aspects of Nonpsychotic Disorders, Jerusalem.

PART I

INNOVATIONS

Section A: Community care for patients with psychotic disorders

Editors' commentary

The three chapters that follow are concerned with programs for the care and management in community settings of individuals with chronic psychotic disorders. The first (Chap. 2), by Mary Ann Test, presents the theoretical and research bases of community care programs for psychotic patients, and provides a general description of the community program for the chronically, severely mentally ill which she and Dr Leonard Stein of the University of Wisconsin developed in Madison, Wisconsin. In the second (Chap. 3) by Dr Julian Leff, Director of the Team for Assessment of Psychiatric Services in the North East Thames Regional Health Authority, London, discusses considerations for community care programs. The third (Chap. 4), by Dr John Hoult, recent Regional Consultant for Mental Health to the Department of Health, New South Wales, Australia, details the problems involved in extending the community care model developed by Stein and Test in Wisconsin on a system-wide basis throughout New South Wales.

There are a number of points to bear in mind while reading these chapters. First, successful models for community care of the severely, chronically mentally ill take into account such patients' ongoing, chronic vulnerabilities. The aim of community care is not cure, but rather ongoing, long-term management. Seriously mentally ill patients who are under the supervision of community care programs do better and display higher levels of functioning than patients in more traditional programs, even though they are not cured.

Providing for such patients in community settings poses formidable problems. Programs must be comprehensive and co-ordinated, including medical, psycho-social, vocational, educational, housing, transportation, and recreational services.

To do this, it is necessary to co-ordinate efforts across levels of government and among community agencies that have never had to work together in the past. Moreover, a clear definition of responsibility is required and care providers need to realize that patient's gains may take many months or even a year, and that support needs to be maintained indefinitely.

In an asylum, the facets of patient care—feeding, clothing, housing, entertaining, employing, and treating them—take place under a single organizational umbrella, funded through a single budget, and administered by a single organization. Community care requires that all these services be provided in an environment with no coherent organization to provide them. In effect, community care has to do everything that any asylum does for the patient, but in an environment where no single person or organization is in charge, with funding coming from multiple sources, with an array of free-standing, autonomous public and private agencies, and jurisdictions that crosscut all levels of government from local to federal.

2

Theoretical and research bases of community care programs

Mary Ann Test & Robert Scott

During the past decade, in the United States and in certain other advanced industrial societies, efforts have been under way to care for persons with severe, chronic psychotic disorders in the community. This approach is being tried in communities of every kind, ranging from large metropolitan areas, to medium- and small-sized urban settings, to rural areas. In general, those responsible for initiating and running such programs are enthusiastic about them. Proponents believe that community care programs in which chronic, severely mentally ill persons are provided with support systems which enable them to cope with daily life outside institutions, and rehabilitation services to limit their social disability, offer a hopeful, cost-effective alternative to the traditional model of treatment involving institutionalization and aftercare.

There is growing evidence from research studies that this optimism is well founded. To date there have been about ten controlled studies which show that a community-based approach to care and management of persons with severe, chronic psychotic disorders allows such individuals to live in freedom in the community, often with fewer relapses and sometimes with less social dysfunction than occurs among similar persons cared for in traditional approaches which rely on institutions (Reviewed and described by Braun et al., 1981, Kiesler, 1982; Test, 1984; Stein & Test, 1980; Test et al., 1985).

These controlled studies share a number of common features. In every case the researchers dealt with severely, chronically impaired mental patients seeking admission to a psychiatric hospital. Such patients were then randomly assigned to two treatment conditions: (a) The usual approach to care involving progressive in-hospital treatment followed by unintensive aftercare; or (b) some version of a community care approach to treatment. Researchers compared the outcomes associated with the treatment condition in which persons were not admitted to hospitals, but were instead treated in community care programs, with the treatment-condition in which patients were assigned to traditional care programs.

The findings of these studies are clear and consistent. Patients randomly assigned to programs which followed a community care model, when compared with those in the hospital-assigned comparison groups, subsequently showed markedly reduced time in institutions; often fewer symptoms and more time between relapses; and, where measured, greater satisfaction with life. In those community programs in which patients received direct assistance in instrumental and social functioning, community-treated patients revealed more favourable psychosocial functioning than those in the traditional care programs. Where economic analyses have been done, they show that a community approach to care and treatment is no more costly than hospitalization, and under certain conditions can be less costly. Patients in community care programs are also found to be no greater a burden to their families or the community than those in hospitals. Finally, the studies also show that these positive results persist for as long as patients remain active clients of community care programs. The evidence suggests that there is a sharp decline in positive functioning when patients leave the community care programs.

The evidence from this 'alternatives to the mental hospital' research, and from a more broadly defined body of community care literatures strongly supports the conclusion that there now exists a means to allow persons suffering from chronic, severe mental illness to live in freedom in the community.

Successful programs of community care are guided by several common principles. They recognize that their clients are continuously vulnerable to even mild or moderate stress, exacerbating psychotic symptoms and resulting in frequent episodes of acute illness. Such persons are engaged in an on-going struggle to accomplish the basic tasks necessary for daily living and most are notably deficient in basic social skills. Given this situation, the programs aim to provide more than just treatment of acute episodes; they offer long-term life support and rehabilitation that is continuous, comprehensive, and intensive. In such programs, community care is not viewed as a cure for chronic mental illness; instead, it is conceived as a method for providing on-going special assistance to severely ill persons, many of whom may never get completely well. Community care programs based on these principles have shown that such persons can live openly in the community as long as they are provided with a life support system to help them cope with their illness and the tasks and routines of daily living in the community, and rehabilitation services to limit social disabilities accompanying their illness.

Effective community care programs share a number of treatment guidelines in common. Obviously, all such programs place top priority on treating patients in the community rather than in hospitals. In order to do this, community-based services must be intensive and comprehensive in nature. In other words, an effective community support system must include provision for crisis intervention, activities of daily living, housing, employment, financial assistance, medical care, mental health care, and social and recreational activities. These and other components of a comprehensive community support system must be tightly integrated and coordinated, with responsibility clearly fixed, in order to ensure continuity of service and to avoid confusion and fragmentation.

Some community care programs also emphasize educating patients about the nature of their illnesses and how to manage them. Patients are taught about the medications they take and how and when they should be taken, and to understand what will happen if they stop taking them. Patients also learn how to manage relapses when these occur and how to deal with ensuing symptoms which are socially disruptive.

Patients who are clients of community care programs require support and instruction with such activities of daily life as finding and maintaining housing, finding proper medical care, shopping for food and preparing it, structuring their time, participating in recreational activities, etc. Finally, they need to acquire and learn how to implement the skills needed to function effectively at work, in social settings, and for living in general.

These services must be organized so that they can be delivered in ways that will reach patients, and that are appropriate to their characteristics. In general, persons who are severely disabled mentally do not usually request assistance when they encounter difficulties, or indeed, even perceive that difficulties are occurring. For this reason, staff members must be assertive in reaching out to patients, seeking defaulters out where they live and work, and helping them in these settings to ensure they are coping well. Treatment programs must be individually tailored and organized in a way that leads to preventing problems arising rather than merely reacting to them after they occur.

Finally, a community support system must extend beyond patients to include their families and their communities as well. Family and community members must be assisted to enable them to deal with the problems posed to them by mentally ill relatives and must be educated about the nature of mental illness to understand what may and may not be expected from such patients in the way of social functioning.

Few community support systems offer comprehensive services. Currently, in most communities there is no single entity capable of doing the entire job. If community care is to be effective, it is essential that responsibility for the care and treatment of patients rests with a single entity.

The community care program developed by Stein & Test in Madison, Wisconsin provides one example of how a program of community care is organized and functions. In this program there is a core team of 15 staff members who provide services for the 120 patients enrolled in it. This team of staff have a clearly designated responsibility for the enrolled patients and are held accountable for seeing to it that all needs of these patients are adequately addressed. Members of the team understand that the buck stops with them, and not somewhere else. They may not transfer responsibility for the treatment or supervision of patients to others. Members of the core team plan and monitor treatment plans for each patient and are also responsible for delivering most of the required services themselves. Staff do not wait to be contacted, but instead take responsibility for reaching out to contact patients and those around them in order to make sure that things are running smoothly. For example, members of the team might contact employers on a daily basis to ensure that certain patients have shown up for work, and visit the patients' place of residence to determine if problems are occurring. Each patient is closely monitored to check that they are taking medication, showing up for work, functioning adequately at home and elsewhere. In order to do this, staff must spend most of their time not in the office but where the patients are. Treatment plans are reviewed daily and changed as necessary. Collaboration with patients in treatment planning and implementation is stressed. Staff also deal with crises, supporting patients during crises and following them up as the episode abates.

This approach to the care and treatment of mental patients must be co-ordinated, assertive, and comprehensive. Figure 2.1 portrays the model of community support that has been implemented in the Madison experiment. Overall, the experience of this program indicates that, if patients are provided with proper life supports and rehabilitation services, it is possible for them to remain in the community and enjoy a degree of freedom and quality of life that is preferable to life inside mental institutions.

While it is true that the number of communities in which such programs have developed is growing, it is also the case that with rare exceptions, implementation of the community-based approach to care has not occurred on a widespread basis. In part, this is because most communities have barriers to implementation of such programs. For example, there are serious fiscal barriers. Third-party payment schemes are not organized in a way that readily facilitates the goals of community care. The fiscal incentives are to institutionalize patients, not to provide them with care as outpatients in the community. In addition, where outpatient services are supported through third party payment, such support tends to be for individual, one-to-one encounters between patients and therapists, and not for provision of social and rehabilitation services.

The fragmented organization of services at the community level is another major barrier to implementing community care programs. The various components

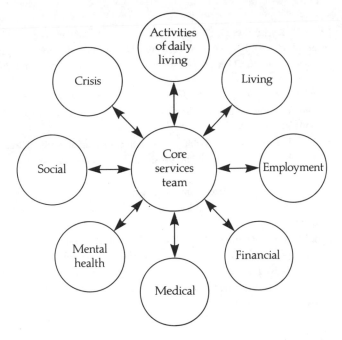

Fig. 2.1. Community Support System.

are a hodge podge of unrelated federal, state, and local governmental programs superimposed on an equally unco-ordinated network of private services. As a result, there is neither a fixed point of responsibility for the individual patient, nor an authority by which to establish this responsibility.

Finally, there are serious barriers within the mental health professions themselves to community care. By and large, professionals prefer to play the roles for which they have been trained and to support the models which favour the *status quo* over change and experimentation. Doing what works can entail such a radical departure from the past, requiring professionals to work together in ways that are so different from what they have been trained to do, that professionals often resist efforts to move the care of the mentally ill in the direction of a community support model.

These considerations notwithstanding, the overall picture is not altogether bleak. If one realizes that a community care approach to the care and management of severe mental disorders is really quite new – having been in operation in the United States for little more than a decade; that the evidence grows that it can and does work effectively; that it is being adopted in many areas of our society, particularly in nonurban areas; and that major Foundations, such as the Robert Wood Johnson Foundation are now providing significant funding for it, then this provides encouragement to move forward in the community care arena.

References

Braun, P., Kockansky, G., Shapiro, R., Greenberg, S., Gudeman, J. E., Johnson, S. & Shore, M. F. (1981). Overview: Deinstitutionalization of psychiatric patients: a critical review of outcome studies. *American Journal of Psychiatry*, **138**, 736–49.

Kiesler, C. A. (1982). Mental hospitals and alternative care: Noninstitutionalization as potential public policy for mental patients. *American Pyschologist*, **37**, 349–60.

Stein, L. I. & Test, M. A. (1980). Alternative to mental hospital treatment: I. Conceptual model, treatment program, and clinical evaluation. *Archives of General Psychiatry*, **37**, 392–7.

Test, M. A., (1984). Community support programs. In (A. S. Belack, ed.) *Schizophrenia: Treatment, Management, Rehabilitation*. New York: Grune and Stratton.

Test, M. A., Knoedler, W. H. & Allness, D. J. (1985). The long term treatment of young schizophrenics in a community support program. In Stein, L. I. & Test, M. A., eds) *The Training in Community Living Model: A Decade of Experience*. New Directions for Mental Health Services, no. 26. San Francisco: Jossey-Bass.

3

Maintenance (management) of people with long-term psychotic illness

Julian Leff

My experience in this field derives from three sources: (a) my clinical responsibility for a small number of admission and long-stay beds in a large psychiatric hospital (Friern) in North London, which serve an area in central London called Bloomsbury, (b) my position as director of the Team for Assessment of Psychiatric Services (TAPS) set up by the North East Thames Regional Health Authority to evaluate their policy of closing two psychiatric hospitals, Friern and Claybury, and replacing them with district-based services, and (c) my research studies of therapeutic intervention in the families of schizophrenic patients.

Each of these endeavours has brought me face to face with the impediments hindering the care of people with chronic psychiatric illnesses. In this paper I will devote some space to these in discussing the various innovations that are being introduced.

Before considering the care and treatment of people with chronic psychiatric illnesses, it is essential to contrast those currently in the community with those remaining in psychiatric hospitals, as their needs may be quite distinct.

Characteristics of chronic psychiatric patients

At any time, the differences between chronic patients in psychiatric hospitals and those in the community depend on the history of the admission and discharge policies of the institutions concerned. Where institutions have operated a conservative discharge policy, long-term inpatients will differ markedly from those living in the community. Institutions with a vigorous discharge policy will have settled many very disabled patients in the community, and there will be more of a continuum between those inside and outside the hospital. One of the research

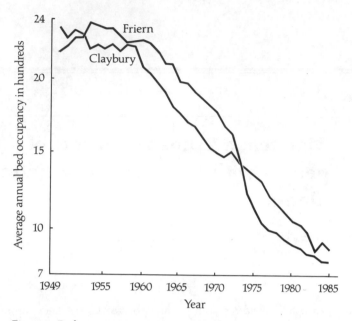

Fig. 3.1. Bed occupancy in Friern and Claybury hospitals 1949–1985.

activities of TAPS is a baseline assessment of the 1000 long-stay (more than one year) nondemented patients in Friern and Claybury Hospitals. The assessments on the whole sample have now been completed, and indicate that the patients in the two hospitals have very similar patterns of disability (NETRHA, 1988).

In fact, as is evident from Figure 3.1, both hospitals have experienced a dramatic and steady decline in bed occupancy over the past 30 years. Friern has declined from a peak of 2373 in 1953 to 786 in 1985, while Claybury's peak was in 1949 at 2336 and its 1985 figure is 864. This difference in current bed occupancy is reflected in a larger number of long-stay nondemented patients in Claybury, 555 compared with 444 in Friern. Since the two hospitals serve catchment areas of similar size, these differences in numbers of long-stay patients suggest the operation of different discharge policies.

Chronic psychiatric patients in hospital
In 1983, in response to the publicly announced decision to close the two hospitals, a census of all the current patients in Friern Hospital was mounted. This was conducted by the medical and nursing staff of the hospital, and yielded information of considerable value for planning community services. We can draw on these data (abstracted from the 1983 Friern Survey (unpublished)) to gain a clearer picture of the patients in the hospital.

Table 3.1. *1983 Friern Survey: symptoms of schizophrenia and duration of stay.*

	Duration of stay			
	< 1 year	1–5 years	5–10 years	> 10 years
Hallucinations	34%	40%	39%	36%
Delusions	55%	63%	50%	36%
Annual exacerbations	NA	63%	58%	48%

Diagnosis is not always easy to establish, particularly for patients admitted several decades previously. However, applying the best diagnosis available, 53% of the total population of 849 inpatients suffered from schizophrenia, 23% from dementia, 11% from affective disorder, and the remaining 13% from a miscellany of other disorders. For the purpose of this paper, we are particularly interested in the long-stay patients. Of the 365 patients who had been in hospital for more than five years, 74% were diagnosed as schizophrenic. It is important to note, though, that 5% of this group suffered from an affective disorder, which can occasionally lead to as poor an outcome as schizophrenia.

It might be thought that these long-stay schizophrenic patients, the residue of custodial practices, are 'burnt-out' cases. The data in Table 3.1 shows that this is not so. Staff were asked to judge whether patients were actively hallucinating or harboured delusions (even if the patients denied them on questioning), and also whether they experienced at least one exacerbation of florid symptoms each year, sufficiently severe to require a change in treatment.

It appears that hallucinations are experienced by a third or more of schizophrenic patients regardless of length of stay. By contrast, delusions do seem to recede over time, once the first year is past. Florid exacerbations are still affecting half of the patients after ten years in hospital, dispelling the notion of 'burn-out', and indicating that, if such patients are transferred to the community, they will continue to require skilled attention. It is evident that many of the schizophrenic patients remaining in psychiatric hospitals are still experiencing delusions and hallucinations despite years, or even decades, of neuroleptic medication. It is known that nearly 10% of patients presenting with an acute attack of schizophrenia fail to respond to neuroleptic drugs and are left with florid symptoms despite continuing medication (Leff & Wing, 1971; Leff *et al.* 1987). In the past, the great majority of these unfortunate people inevitably become long-term inpatients. They form a substantial proportion of the residual long-stay population of psychiatric hospitals, and constitute a considerable challenge to community care. The problems posed by such patients and the attempts made to tackle them will occupy much of this paper.

Some patients who are apparently free of florid psychiatric symptoms continue to be cared for in hospital for other reasons. In particular, we have been impressed in the course of our assessments by the problem of multiple handicaps. In addition to a psychiatric condition, now quiescent, patients are found to suffer from personality disorders, alcoholism, sensory defects such as deafness, and a variety of physical ailments, including diabetes, heart failure, chronic bronchitis, and renal disease. These latter are a consequence of the elderly nature of the long-stay population, and necessitate considerable expertise for their treatment and management. It is seldom recognized that the medical staff in psychiatric hospitals function as general practitioners for the patients, and that the nursing staff keep a close eye on their physical condition. These important functions need to be replicated in the community.

Chronic psychiatric patients in the community
This population can be divided into two groups: those currently supported by established services, and those unsupported.
Supported community patients
Supported patients consist of individuals who have never spent long periods in psychiatric hospitals, but who would have done so in the custodial era (the potential 'new long-stay'), and patients discharged from psychiatric hospitals after long periods of inpatient care. The potential new long-stay are of great interest, since they constitute a test of the effectiveness of a community-based service in preventing institutionalism. This is a difficult group to identify precisely, since they are defined hypothetically as those who *would have become* long-stay under the old custodial system. Nevertheless, they must form a proportion of patients included in experimental programs like those of Stein & Test (1980) and Hoult (1986). A group of such patients was studied by Sturt, Wykes & Creer (1982) in the London borough of Camberwell. They were defined as any individual, aged 18 or above, who was resident in or attending one of the community psychiatric day or residential units and who had been in contact with some psychiatric service (including outpatient clinics) for a year or more. The patients not in residential care were evenly distributed among the following types of household: living with a spouse or cohabitee, living with a parent or other relative, living alone or sharing a flat or house. This finding stresses the important role that relatives play in supporting such patients in the community. In Test's programs, staff provide support to family members who are involved with the patient, even though the patient may not be living with them, while Hoult's crisis teams inform relatives about mental illness and give them guidance.

In the group of patients included in the study of Sturt *et al.*, just over one-quarter of the group had no daytime occupation, and this was equally true of men and women. The series contained a large number of patients with a very long history of service contact: nearly three-quarters had first contacted a psychiatric service, and two-thirds had first been admitted more than ten years previously. Half the group were given a diagnosis of schizophrenia, and nearly half of the patients were handicapped by some quite serious physical disability, including epilepsy, sensory defects, hypertension, heart disease and diabetes.

The picture that emerges from this survey is of a group of people chronically handicapped by both psychiatric and physical illnesses. In many ways they resemble the long-stay patients we are assessing in Friern and Claybury Hospitals, indicating that they are indeed a similar population for whom chronic hospitalization has been successfully avoided. However, the prevention of hospitalization has not automatically guaranteed psychiatric health. There is confirmatory evidence from other studies (Johnstone *et al.*, 1981; Westermeyer, 1980) that patients with chronic schizophrenia who are maintained in the community exhibit a similar range of psychological and social deficits to those staying in hospital for long periods. Whether these are an inevitable consequence of the illness, or whether they could be avoided by innovatory methods of care, remains an open question.

Unsupported community patients

Undoubtedly a small number of chronically mentally ill people lose touch with the relevant services, but manage to survive in the community in reasonable circumstances, possibly through the support of relatives or friends (Johnstone *et al.*, 1984). However, the great majority of such people rapidly drift into a vagrant lifestyle, shuttling between living rough, brief spells in prison, and short admissions to psychiatric facilities. They never receive adequate treatment for their florid symptoms, and are not usually kept long enough in a psychiatric facility for any form of rehabilitation to be attempted. They tend to congregate in inner-city areas, particularly where railway termini and bus depots exist. Bloomsbury, wherein my own clinical responsibilities lie, contains three major railway termini, as a consequence of which 20% of admissions to Friern from this district are of no fixed abode or from outside the catchment area. This contrasts with a figure of 4% for the other three districts served by Friern. If it were possible to calculate the number of vagrant psychotic people in a country, this would provide a revealing index of the relative adequacy of community care in that country as a whole. In the current service, vagrant psychotic people are dealt with by buck-passing, an inhumane and, in the long run, a costly evasion of responsibility. Methods of caring for and treating them need to be developed in the context of community-based service, and will be discussed later.

Innovations in care and treatment

Having discussed the characteristics of chronic psychiatric patients in and out of hospital, we can proceed to consider innovations in their care and treatment, both in operation and still to be introduced. It is convenient to categorize these according to their function: psychiatric patients like everyone else need a place to live, some form of work-like activity, and something to do in their leisure hours.

A place to live

When long-stay patients first began to be discharged from psychiatric hospitals in the early 1950s, many of them went to live on their own. This was possible because the least disabled patients were naturally chosen first for discharge. Watt & Buglass (1966) compared all the nondemented long-stay patients discharged from a psychiatric hospital between 1954 and 1961 with those remaining as inpatients. They found that 45% of those discharged were judged as having no symptoms compared with only 16% of those remaining ($P < 0.001$). Some patients returned to their relatives, but this could be a mixed blessing, since if relatives were critical of the patient or overinvolved, a relapse and readmission was very likely (Brown et al., 1962, 1972; Vaughn & Leff, 1976). As discharge continued at a steady rate (see Fig. 3.1) the hospitals were depleted of patients who could readily live on their own, and staff were faced with the need to introduce innovatory methods of care for the more disabled patients. A variety of these had developed at an astronomical pace. Carpenter (1978) reported that in the United States only two such facilities existed in 1950; by 1960, 40 halfway houses were identified, by 1969, 128, and by 1973, 209. Brown (1985) estimated that currently throughout the United States close to one million mentally disabled persons live in nursing and boarding homes.

Group homes

The degree of supervision in such accommodation varies considerably from visits by staff once a week or less to a continuous presence, with staffing levels equal to those on acute admission wards. One of the earliest innovations was co-operative or group homes, in which a small number of patients lived together forming a household with no resident staff. It became the practice to set up such groups on a trial basis in accommodation in the hospital grounds. Substitutions were often necessary for patients who did not fit in during the trial period. Once the group achieved stability, it moved out into accommodation in the community. Fairly intense supervision was maintained by staff initially, but this was gradually reduced to approximately weekly visits. Some of the earliest experiments of this nature were linked with schemes to provide the residents with paid work (e.g. Fairweather et al., 1969). Admirable as these endeavours were, they never swept the country, either in the United Kingdom or the United States, because of a scarcity of patients with sufficient ability to staff them. The aims of most group homes are much more modest: usually some residents attend for sheltered work activities daily, while the others carry out the domestic chores necessary to run the home. It is in the nature of group homes that they cannot sustain residents who do not pull their weight, by working either outside or inside the home. While such homes are still being established from time to time in the United Kingdom, their heyday is over, as the great majority of patients with sufficient ability have already been accommodated.

Landlords

The next level of intensity of supervision involves a nonprofessional person or persons living in the same accommodation as the patients. This is exemplified by landlord-supervised apartments. The landlord usually lives in an adjacent dwelling and assumes some responsibility for ensuring that patients get up in time for their daily program and are adequately fed and housed. It is possible to make a comfortable living from this form of care, and in the United Kingdom psychiatric nurses have begun to set up their own boarding homes, sometimes accommodating as many as ten former inpatients This is considerably more profitable than working as a state-employed nurse. However, some individuals have continued in their full-time nursing jobs, which casts doubt on the amount of supervision they are able to give their residents. There are clearer advantages for such establishments to be run by a psychiatric nurse rather than a lay landlord, but on the other hand there is a danger of institutional attitudes engendered in the hospital staff being carried over into the residential environment. Another concern is that legislation has not yet caught up with these developments in the United Kingdom and there is no statutory requirement for any kind of inspection of homes containing four or fewer residents.

The widespread use in the United States of board and care homes and nursing homes must be mentioned here. Severe criticisms have been levelled, for example by Brown (1985), at this practice which appears to be maintained by expediency and the profit motive rather than by careful planning for patients' needs. Brown estimates that the annual turnover of board and care homes has reached 16 billion dollars, a commercial venture of such magnitude that it has attracted the attention of the Mafia.

A similar scheme, but on a much smaller scale, was attempted in the United Kingdom. For some years, patients were discharged from long-stay care to live in seaside boarding houses. These were relatively cheap, and patients were welcome as a source of income out of season. However, no attempt was made to provide any activities for the patients, and the pathetic images of these unfortunate people trudging the rain-swept streets of derelict seaside towns were used by the media to provoke a public scandal. As a result, this form of care is rarely utilized.

Foster families

A more personal form of supervision is provided by foster families. This is not a recent innovation, since families in Gheel, Belgium, have taken mentally ill people into their homes for 600 years (Airing, 1974), and a similar scheme was set up in Aro village, Nigeria, by Lambo over 30 years ago. However, in the United States and the United Kingdom, this form of care has become widespread only recently. Budson (1983) reports that in the United States the Veterans' Administration has relied more heavily on foster care than the state systems. Up to four residents may be placed in one foster home, and the family providing care is supervised by a visiting social worker from the referring institution. In the United Kingdom the degree of integration of the patient into the family varies from occupation of a separate apartment in the same house as the family, to sharing everything with the family but a bedroom. The latter arrangement has the advantage of surrounding the patient with a supportive group of people, but there are possible disadvantages too. Our recent experience of working with one foster family who were hosting two schizophrenic patients, has shown us that high Expressed Emotion (EE) attitudes can be detected in foster parents. They also seem to have the same deleterious effect on the outcome of schizophrenia as has been found with parents, spouses, and other family members (Leff & Vaughn, 1985). This suggests that either a more rigorous screening procedure should be applied to potential foster parents, or else specialized forms of support should be offered to foster families hosting psychiatric patients.

Hostels

Hostels provide a more professional form of care than landlords or foster families, although some hostel wardens, particularly in establishments set up by voluntary bodies, may not have a background in the caring professions. However, most organizations responsible for hostels now provide some form of training for wardens. The Richmond Fellowship, a voluntary body formed in England but now with international ramification, is a good example of an organization which takes the training of its wardens very seriously and runs intensive courses.

Whatever the background of the carer taking responsibility for a resident who has a chronic psychiatric illness, he or she needs adequate training for the tasks involved. This has rarely been provided for landlords or foster families, even though it is manifestly unrealistic to assume that they have an intuitive knowledge of the best way to help psychiatric patients. Furthermore, any care-giver who is in regular contact with the patients requires emotional support from an experienced professional. In the absence of this, a high rate of burn-out can be anticipated. Hoult claims that burn-out is not a serious problem in the New South Wales project. However, this was probably achieved by a redeployment of the original research staff to run new services in other areas. Burn-out develops when staff work for long periods of time with chronic psychotic patients, where progress is inevitably at a snail's pace. This issue will be taken up later in discussing the co-ordination of community facilities.

'Hospital-hostels' or 'Wards in the community'?

The forms of sheltered accommodation considered above are suitable for patients with a wide range of disabilities, but would not provide adequate care for many of the long-stay patients still remaining in psychiatric hospitals. In particular, patients with persistent florid symptoms, or with pronounced negative symptoms, require more intensive supervision and help than could reasonably be expected from landlords, foster families, or hostel wardens. The extent of their clinical and social disabilities has been revealed by a spate of psychiatric hospital surveys in the United Kingdom, stimulated by a vigorously pursued government policy of closure (e.g. Levene, Donaldson & Brandon, 1985). Furthermore, it has become apparent that 'new long-stay' patients are accumulating in each district in the United Kingdom, requiring about 40 beds per 100,000 population (18 beds for those under 65 years of age) and that these patients have disabilities of a similar level of severity to the old long-stay remaining in psychiatric hospitals (Wykes, 1982).

A number of solutions to this problem have been put into effect in the United Kingdom, while others are on the verge of implementation. In three places, London, Southampton, and Manchester, a specialized facility has been created specifically for the chronically mentally ill. The first to be established was the 'hospital-hostel' at the Maudsley Hospital in 1977. It consists of a converted Victorian house sited in the grounds of the hospital, but fronting the main road. It was intended to provide 'a domestic-scale environment for new long-stay patients who would otherwise be living on hospital wards with sufficient staff to ensure that they received a fair-share of social contact and supervision' (Wykes, 1982). Places for 14 patients were provided, with seven double bedrooms. The nurse:patient ratio is one to one, and there is also a half-time clinical psychologist, a full-time domestic help, and an occupational therapy aide. The same basic services are provided as in hospital wards, including meals. Most of the residents found sheltered occupation in the Maudsley Hospital or nearby. However, two remained on the hostel-ward during the day because they were too unco-operative and disruptive to use other day settings. Nurses from the hostel-ward accompany some of the more disabled residents to their day activity. The front door is locked for two 2-hour periods in the morning and afternoon to prevent residents returning who should be at work. It was initially hoped that some residents would become less dependent and would move to local authority hostels, group homes or other suitable accommodation. By December 1980, two hostel-ward patients had been discharged and plans were made for six others to move into a group home. One of the discharged patients committed suicide three months later, while the other was still living with his family at the time of the report.

The Maudsley hospital-hostel differs from conventional wards for the long-stay in its architecture, the high staff:patient ratio, and the care taken by the psychologist to plan programmes for each resident. However, it relies heavily on the hospital for back-up services and is in no way integrated into the community.

The Southampton hostel differs most obviously from the Maudsley facility in being sited away from the hospital. It consists of two adjacent houses in a terrace a few minutes' walk from the district general hospital, which contains a psychiatric unit. However, in other respects it is very similar: a high nurse:patient ratio, the assistance of a psychologist, and an occupational therapist, and domestic help. In fact there is a full-time cook, who plans menus and prepares meals from raw materials provided by the hospital. Most of the residents are quite severely disabled and contribute little to the running of the hostel; some of them help in preparing vegetables for cooking. There is an attempt to promote a domestic atmosphere, but official notices on the walls, including in the bedrooms, undermine this. The facility is best described as a long-stay ward which has been sited in the community and has the benefit of a high professional input.

The Manchester hostel goes further than the other two in attempting to increase the autonomy and independence of the residents. Known as Douglas House it is situated in a socially desirable neighbourhood about a mile from the main hospital campus. The hostel opened in 1982 and was set up to provide an appropriate environment for the 20 patients from the catchment area of the district general hospital who had stayed on the psychiatric wards for more than 6 months. The maximum number of residents is 12, and there is a complement of nine nurses. A psychologist advises on a programme for each resident, and a speech therapist organizes a group aimed at improving communication skills. Where Douglas House differs radically from the other two hostels is in its guiding philosophy, namely that 'living skills such as choosing menus, shopping for food, cooking, serving food, washing up, cleaning the house, doing one's laundry, household maintenance, and gardening are in fact *much more appropriate re-enabling activities* for patients who have spent much time in hospital than those they are likely to be offered in a day center, workshop, or occupational therapy department' (Goldberg *et al.*, 1985). The nurses are given a weekly allowance by the hospital with which to buy food and other consumables, and some residents participate in shopping and preparing meals. The tailor-made program for each resident focuses on self-care, domestic skills, social skills, and special problems. Points and bonuses are gained by achieving targets and are exchanged for money at a weekly pay-out meeting. Of the 16 patients who have been residents of Douglas House, three were judged as failures, while two have moved on to less sheltered accommodation in the community.

These three forms of accommodation attempt to provide a sheltered environment for chronically ill patients, while minimizing the risk of in-stitutionalism. Only Douglas House appears to have created an environment that differs substantially from a ward in a psychiatric hospital. Hoult reports that hospital-hostels represent the most sheltered end of the range of accommodation provided in the New South Wales program.

More radical solutions are currently being considered, some of them in relation to the proposed closure of Friern and Claybury Hospitals. A strategy common to many of the districts involved is to acquire residential housing, convert it into individual bedrooms or self-contained flats, and move groups of long-stay patients into the converted houses. The self-contained flats are obviously intended for the more able patients, while at the other end of the dependence scale, some of the houses with single bedrooms would have numbers of staff in attendance throughout the day and night. I am most conversant with the plans from the Bloomsbury district of London for which I have some clinical responsibility. The planning is based on a number of guidelines, which stem from a desire to create as normal an environment as possible and to avoid institutionalism. They are as follows:

1. single bedrooms in domestic style and scale building. Residents will be living in the accommodation for many years, if not for the rest of their lives. There is no reason why they should have to share their bedroom with another person. People with chronic schizophrenia especially need privacy. Converting residential housing ensures that the structure will be as domestic as possible.

2. space giving the option of socializing or privacy. Residents need somewhere within the house to which they can withdraw if they wish to be alone, as well as areas in which social activities are encouraged.

3. a sheltered garden. Whatever their deficiencies, the old psychiatric hospitals at least provided bountiful outdoor space in which disturbed patients could pace about unhindered, and could work off their restlessness. Land is too expensive in cities to recreate such spaces, but at least a garden ought to be included if possible. It needs to be sheltered from the public gaze to ensure privacy for the residents, many of whom are likely to have obvious peculiarities which attract the attention of the curious. The other advantage of a garden is that it can be used to provide horticultural activities for some of the residents, as in Douglas House.

4. a sheltered work facility providing for a range of abilities, within easy reach of the residence. This guideline runs contrary to the principle behind the activities organized in Douglas House. Whereas the latter have an advantage in providing a potential occupation for each resident, they entail the serious disadvantage of confining the residents within the same building in which they sleep. One of the main criticisms levelled by Goffman (1961) at total institutions was that they provided for all activities – sleep, work, leisure – under one roof. A sheltered work place separate from the hostel ensures that the residents meet a different group of people in a different milieu and that they pass through a normal environment to reach it. However, it should not be so far away as to constitute a barrier for the more disabled residents: either within walking distance or a single bus ride away is the limit.

5. the facility should be integrated with the local community. A common fate for such hostels is to become isolated outposts of the psychiatric hospital, within the community but not part of it. In order for full integration to occur, the public has to go beyond passive acceptance to active involvement with the residents. This will be discussed further in the section on leisure activities, but it is appropriate to deal here with the issue of informing and educating the public.

Within the planning teams responsible for the reprovision of services supplied by Friern and Claybury Hospitals, there exists a wide variety of opinion on informing the public, ranging from the view that it is best to purchase a house clandestinely and slip the residents in unnoticed, to a stated policy of open government with full public consultation. There are no studies of the relative effectiveness of these various approaches, but my own preference is for providing the public with as much information as possible. This policy runs the risk of encountering fierce opposition to the siting of a hostel in the neighbourhood, and indeed this has already arisen numerous times. Goldberg *et al.* (1985) record that the plans to open Douglas House caused grave disquiet in the neighbourhood, but that a public meeting arranged by the Community Health Council won over the objectors. The Richmond Fellowship, a voluntary organization, makes door-to-door house calls in the neighbourhood to explain their plans to set up a hostel and to answer queries. Only one of their many hostels has been blocked by local opposition.

My view is that public meetings attract those neighbours most vociferously antagonistic to the proposed facility and that there is likely to be a silent majority of nonattenders who are at least neutral, if not capable of being won over by a suitable educational program. Therefore TAPS proposed to conduct a house-to-house survey of public attitudes before any hostel was established. It was considered that the knowledge gained would identify those with positive attitudes who could be recruited to help the integration of the residents, as well as indicating the kind of educational efforts required to influence those with negative attitudes. Two of the district planning teams would not permit the survey to be conducted because they feared it would inflame a public already expressing antagonism to a proposed hostel. Fortunately, Haringey district approved the survey, which has now been completed.

It has to be recognized that the anxieties of the public are not entirely without foundation; not of course, their fears of violence and sexual misdemeanours, but those relating to the nuisance value of the residents. Of the 16 residents of Douglas House, the behaviour of three caused public offence (Goldberg *et al.*, 1985). Two were temporarily banned from the local pub: one because of persistent obscenities accompanied by regurgitating his food in front of other customers, the other because of persistent importuning for cigarettes or a coke. Another resident was asked to leave a local café after she was incontinent. As the process of running down the psychiatric hospitals makes increasing inroads into the population of the most disabled patients, it is inevitable that peculiar and frankly offensive behaviour will become more common in public places. A combination of two approaches is probably indicated: psychological methods of extinguishing the undesirable behaviour, and education of the public to reduce their anxieties about expatients of psychiatric hospitals. The former has already proved its worth, while the latter is in its infancy. The mass media should certainly be utilized as was done in Italy.

6. Residents must be involved in decisions about their home and their lives. The first decision is where they are to live on leaving hospital, and they should certainly be consulted on this, although ambivalent answers may be anticipated from a high proportion of patients. Once settled in accommodation in the community, residents should be involved in choosing the decor of their rooms, in making up menus for the week, and in decisions about the running of the house. These practices are common in therapeutic communities, where they developed as a means of flattening the hierarchy of professional power and status. However, they only filtered through in a diluted form to psychiatric hospitals as a whole. As a consequence, it is difficult for the average psychiatric nurse to share power and authority equally with patients. One solution would be to staff such sheltered accommodation with personnel who have not been trained in psychiatric hospitals. However, as discussed on p. 19, many of the patients currently being considered for discharge suffer from florid psychotic symptoms which need skilled and experienced people to cope with them. A compromise that has been adopted in the United Kingdom is to use housing associations to purchase and run the hostels. These are voluntary organizations, unconnected with the Health Service, that have the added advantage of being able to bid for capital made available by the government for house purchases of a general kind. Trained psychiatric nurses, paid by the local health district, are then employed to staff the hostel, but come under the management of the housing association, which has potentially much more flexibility than the Health Service. Naturally, in this situation nurses have greatly increased independence and autonomy compared with hospital conditions, and they need special training to adapt themselves to it.

Work

Warner (1985) argues that efforts to rehabilitate psychiatric patients are directly related to the demands of the labour market. A boom leads to increased pressure to add disabled patients to the work force. The reverse is certainly true, that in times of high unemployment, as at present in the United Kingdom, a history of prolonged hospitalization or psychiatric treatment makes it virtually impossible for patients to obtain jobs on the open market. Sheltered employment is well developed in psychiatric hospitals in the United Kingdom, in contrast with the United States where employment within hospitals is not allowed. However, there is a dearth of such facilities in the community in Britain. Existing day hospitals and day centres in the United Kingdom do not provide the variety of jobs available in the better psychiatric hospitals, the large size of which is an advantage in this respect. Friern hospital, for example, provides daily paid employment for 120 patients. A sizable proportion of these commute in from accommodation in the community, reflecting the paucity of appropriate extramural facilities.

As already indicated, there was a phase in the run-down of psychiatric hospitals in which patients were placed in sheltered accommodation but no work-like activities were provided. It is now acknowledged by the planners that this was a serious omission. Work fulfils many important needs for the healthy citizen, but additionally, for chronic psychotic patients it is actually therapeutic (Wing & Freudenberg, 1961). When asked directly, patients will often confirm that they are less troubled by auditory hallucinations when they are actively engaged in some task. Current plans link sheltered accommodation with schemes for providing work-like activities.

Most hospital workshops and day centres in the United Kingdom rely on contract work as their mainstay; that is, repetitive assembly or packaging tasks are performed by the patients on materials sent out by private businesses and factories on a contractual basis. Additionally, the more enterprising workshops design and produce their own products, such as soft toys, dolls' house furniture, bird tables and so on. These provide more interesting tasks for patients of above-average ability. However, the bulk of work is contractual and this ensures the financial viability of most workshops. Since contract work is supplied to businesses in the open market, it has to meet deadlines which can only be guaranteed if there is a sufficiently large pool of patients attending the workshop regularly. It is difficult to sustain this kind of activity in a small work place, because a proportion of patients will have unpredictable 'off-days' leading to a fall in production.

Two solutions to this problem have been proposed. One is to set up in each district a large day activities centre, positioned so that it is within easy reach of most, if not all, the sheltered accommodation that is to be established. The other, which dovetails with the first, is to concentrate more on making 'own products' and providing services needed by the local community than on contract work. A good example of this kind of planning is provided by Bloomsbury, in which the day activities centre will be sited in a now-empty nurses' hostel. The building stands on one of the main roads running through the district, close to a large housing estate and to four houses which are being converted into hostels for long-stay patients from Friern Hospital. The building has large rooms on the entrance floor which it is planned to turn into a café. The café will be run by patients who will prepare food under supervision and serve at the tables. It is hoped that the café will attract clientele from the local community. In addition, another large room in the basement may be hired out for functions, such as birthdays and receptions, for which catering could be supplied by the patients. There is also space to house an already established print shop, which is highly successful, employs six or seven patients, and intends to expand. The building has a reasonably sized garden in which vegetables and flowers could be grown for sale. The possibility has been discussed of canvassing the local housing estate to find out what services the residents consider are lacking in the neighbourhood, which might then be supplied by the day activities centre.

In the LINC program in Oregon, contracts have been developed with a number of local employers to provide a range of services, such as housekeeping, gardening and landscaping, and restaurant work (Faulkner *et al.*, 1983).

The aims of the Bloomsbury project are clearly to provide a range of work activities, more varied and hence more interesting than contract work, but still with slots for the most disabled patients. If the café is able to attract local residents, then integration into the community becomes a stronger possibility.

This kind of planning requires entrepreneurial skills, which are not often found among psychiatric staff or professional administrators. The few schemes of this type that have achieved success (e.g. Fairweather *et al.*, 1969) have been promoted by very unusual and enthusiastic individuals. If they are to become widespread, a different method of establishing them needs to be found. It is possible that recruitment of successful businessmen to give advice on a voluntary basis might be an answer. Whatever solutions are found, it is important that the most disabled patients should not be ignored and allowed to remain inactive.

Leisure

My office is in a building immediately opposite the long-stay ward for which I am responsible, which is itself situated in a large Edwardian house, isolated from the rest of the hospital. The 14 men who live in this house all suffer from chronic schizophrenia, and 12 of them are occupied daily in a variety of activities around the hospital. I watch them going out to work and coming back for meals and am always struck by the fact that they walk in Indian file, never closer than ten yards to the next man, despite many of them having lived in close proximity for eight years or more. Their social activity on the ward shows the same distancing from each other. Almost all social interchange is mediated through the single nurse on duty, who initiates conversations and games with the residents. The one exception is an elderly man who has lived in the hospital for 30 years, but remarkably has retained an engaging extroverted manner – he always wishes me a good weekend when I go off on a Friday afternoon. He plays draughts, at which he is expert, with several of the other residents. Wykes (1982) reported that virtually all social activity in the Maudsley hospital-hostel was channelled through the nursing staff.

Social interchange between long-stay patients has such a low profile that it is very difficult for an observer to detect the existence of social bonds. Nevertheless, it is important to make an attempt at this, since it is planning policy in moving patients out of the hospital not to separate friends. Since many long-stay patients are very taciturn, if not mute, it is likely that social bonding is achieved largely by non-verbal behaviour, such as choosing to sit next to a particular person, exchanging cigarettes, or running errands. TAPS researchers administer a Social Network Schedule to patients and staff in order to determine whom the patients consider to be friends. Obviously this cannot be completed for mute or near-mute patients, and in these instances it is our impression that the staff are uncertain who are socially significant persons for the patients. Therefore we have instituted a study of nonverbal and verbal social behaviour in a small sample of long-stay patients in order to test the validity of our questionnaire. It would be clearly impossible to make these observations on a large group, which is what is really needed if the policy of keeping friends together is to be honoured.

Patients living outside of the hospital should have their leisure needs attended to. The staff in sheltered accommodation will certainly continue to perform the social roles nurses fulfil in hospital, but this is not sufficient if patients are to be integrated into the normal community. Furthermore, to avoid the development of a 'total institution', leisure activities should be pursued in a different setting from the hostel. The commonest facility to be provided is a drop-in centre or club for ex-patients. Sometimes these remain open in the evenings and at weekends, when patients are likely to be at a loose end. However, these places are prone to develop an institutional atmosphere, with a small number of healthy staff and a large number of patients, few of whom are socially outgoing. Ideally, patients should be enabled to mix with healthy people in situations where they are in the minority. Regular visits to relatives would help considerably, but many of the long-stay patients have lost touch with their families, who would not welcome a renewal of contact. Sometimes, however, patients are sufficiently improved by discharge to a community setting for their relatives to experience a change of heart.

In the absence of interested family members, it is possible to recruit volunteers to befriend patients. The COPE program in Oregon centres on a social club which is staffed entirely by volunteers from a wide variety of backgrounds. These include church members, student nurses, college students and retired people. Relationships develop between volunteers and patients which extend well beyond the formal daily meeting times (Nathan & Beigel, 1982). The initiative needs to be taken to develop a wide network of volunteers who would befriend even the most disabled of patients. This is not a very rewarding task and requires persistence and enthusiasm. There are plenty of unemployed and retired people who might find that it gives a sense of purpose to their lives. However, volunteering for this kind of role requires a social consciousness which is all too rare. It is probably necessary to introduce teaching in schools which develops an awareness in the pupils of their capacity to help their more unfortunate disabled fellows. Religious organizations, as a matter of course, embody this in their instruction but with the waning of their power and influence, it needs to be adopted by secular teachers.

Vagrants

Vagrant psychotic patients are usually admitted to psychiatric wards from the police, from casualty departments or from voluntary organizations such as the Samaritans and St Mungo's. They are often dirty, smelly, unkempt and ungrateful, and do not wish to stay in hospital. They are commonly allowed to discharge themselves after a short admission or when the legal section they were brought in on expires. This action is often justified by labelling the patient as 'personality disorder', even when delusions and hallucinations are clearly present. This method of dealing with vagrants is short sighted, because they rapidly repeat the cycle of sleeping rough, being picked up by the police, and being readmitted to a psychiatric ward, usually a different one where they are not known, so that the process starts afresh. No community-based service can claim to be comprehensive if it fails to make provision for vagrant psychotic patients.

Our own practice is dominated by vagrants, who form 20% of admissions to Friern Hospital from Bloomsbury. We have had considerable experience with unmedicated schizophrenic patients who have been leading a vagrant life, and we have been surprised at the rapidity with which some of them improve on neuroleptic medication (Leff & Tress, 1986). In others, it takes months before their psychotic symptoms come under pharmacological control. We have found that a high proportion of them shun any attempt at intimacy and become increasingly paranoid if it is forced on them. Some respond to the threat of a more stable relationship with staff or other patients by discharging themselves. However, we have found that if we emphasize to them that we regard them as our responsibility and advise them to contact us when they need help, they usually return to us after a short absence. Some patients have left several times in this manner, before finally settling down in the hospital.

Of course, there is a danger of institutionalizing such patients, so the policy is to pursue an active course of rehabilitation. The great majority of vagrants we admit respond to this, and after one or two years in hospital are transferred to sheltered accommodation linked with day activity.

It appears to us that a relatively lengthy period of active treatment and rehabilitation is essential before the cycle of vagrancy, prison and short-term admissions to hospital can be broken. Community-based programs in large cities must be able to respond to the needs of vagrants, but whether this is possible in the context of current plans for sheltered accommodation and activity remains unclear.

Co-ordination and monitoring

The traditional 'ward round' held on the psychiatric ward of a general hospital or in a psychiatric hospital is an efficient method of co-ordinating a multidisciplinary team, consisting of doctors, nurses, occupational therapists and social workers. Once the focus of care moves into the community, co-ordination poses a considerable problem. One obvious solution is to set up a community mental health centre, which can act as a base for the various professionals involved in the care of chronically ill patients in the community. The community mental health centre movement in the United States has by no means been an unqualified success, and has been heavily criticized by some (e.g. Brown, 1985). The Community Mental Health Centers Act was made law by Congress in 1963. According to Ozarin & Levenson (1967) one of the main tasks of the Centres was the maintenance of chronic patients in the community. However, this demanding and relatively unrewarding job was overtaken in priority by two more glamorous aims, also listed by Ozarin & Levenson: resolution of emotional crises in individuals and families, and early case finding. In fact Brown (1985) states that, instead of supporting chronic patients discharged from psychiatric hospitals, the Centres catered for a completely new clientele comprising people in the general population with minor psychiatric complaints. It is encouraging to learn from Hoult that in New South Wales the attitudes of existing community mental health staff have been changing towards the care of the severely mentally ill as a top priority.

The United Kingdom is on the brink of a country-wide expansion in community mental health centres, which at the moment exist in only a few districts. From the viewpoint of psychiatric hospitals, they are seen primarily as a method of co-ordinating support for chronic patients and monitoring the effectiveness of the service. But there must be a substantial risk that they will develop in the same way as those in the United States. Indeed, an analysis of the first few years of operation of a Community Mental Health Centre in a district of London revealed that about half the referrals were new cases (Fagin, unpublished results). This figure indicates that a major function of the Centre is that of a primary care mental health facility.

The setting-up of such Centres draws professionals out of hospitals and leads to the development of innovatory services. For example, the Centre referred to above was associated with the following novel schemes: psychologists established a District Psychology Service with attachments to the majority of the local large GP practices; psychiatrists developed an *ad hoc* crisis intervention service, with joint home assessments, as well as emergency outpatient clinics based within the local social services departments; community psychiatric nurses began to take direct referrals from primary care settings (Fagin & Purser, unpublished results). It is evident that these exciting developments contribute little to the maintenance of chronic patients in the community. It should be noted that the programs in Madison and New South Wales place a strong emphasis on the community care of this particular clientele. It is easy for such patients to disappear from the ken of the professionals, particularly if they harbour negative attitudes towards the services on offer. One way of ensuring that they remain visible is to establish a case register based in the community mental health centre. This has actually been achieved in the Centre referred to above.

Limited case registers

Comprehensive psychiatric case registers have been in existence for many years and aim to record all contacts with psychiatric hospital services, inpatient and outpatient, made by residents of a defined geographical area. Their usefulness lies in providing a framework for epidemiological studies and for evaluative studies of conventional psychiatric services (e.g. Wing & Hailey, 1972). Because they are comprehensive and include large numbers of patients, it has not been feasible to collect detailed data concerning community facilities such as day centres, day hospitals, community psychiatric nurses and general practitioners. However, with the shift in focus of care from the psychiatric hospital to the district, these facilities assume increasing importance. It is only possible to cover such a wide range of services if the case register is restricted to a particular group of patients. One obvious group on which to concentrate is the chronically mentally ill, since they are bound to be among the heaviest users of community services.

The development of modern computers with disc storage systems has made it possible to set up limited case registers in the community. The one installed in the community mental health centre described above, has already been used to analyse the characteristics of its clients over the years 1984 to 1986 (Fagin, unpublished results). This innovatory practice is likely to spread, resulting in a computer in every community health centre within a district, all being interlinked through a central computer, perhaps located in the district general hospital. If such a network were eventually to cover the whole of the United Kingdom it would become relatively easy to keep track of chronic psychotic patients who wander from district to district, and for the first time to estimate accurately the size of this derelict stage army.

Another major benefit of a limited case register would be the ability to monitor patients' use of a wide range of community services; not just whether they are in contact, but their actual frequency of usage. This would enable case-workers to detect holes in the network of services and to prevent patients from falling through them. It has been pointed out that neglect in psychiatric hospitals eventually leads to public scandals, whereas neglect in the community can easily remain invisible. Data detailed enough for this kind of monitoring could be collected by the key-worker for each patient each time a visit is made. It would be necessary to check how many times the patient had attended a day activity facility, a drop-in centre, the GP, etc since last being seen. These data would be fed into the microprocessor in the community health centre by the key-worker on returning from a batch of visits.

The best way to ensure that this is done conscientiously is to demonstrate the clinical value to the key-workers. A review of the patients maintained on the register should be conducted at regular intervals by a member of staff designated for this task. Printouts would show graphically the pattern of service usage for each patient, and would instantly reveal any gaps. Rather than making one of the clinical staff responsible for reviewing patients on the register, it would be preferable to assign this task to a secretary/administrator, an essential member of the community mental health centre team. This form of case register is now technically feasible and relatively inexpensive, and is likely to become an integral part of most district-based services for chronically ill psychiatric patients.

Utilization of psychiatric hospital sites

The majority of psychiatric hospitals were built on extensive sites, which, with the shrinkage and eventual closure of the hospitals, become available for other uses. The most obvious outcome is for the spare land to be sold for residential or commercial development, and for the capital realized to be ploughed back into community services. However, there are other ways in which the land can be utilized to benefit psychiatric patients. In Italy, it has been the policy to build facilities for the public on land released by the psychiatric hospitals. For example, schools have been erected on these sites, thus bringing healthy children and adults into proximity with the long-stay patients still remaining in the hospital.

The plans for Friern Hospital incorporate a different kind of scheme. Friern serves four health districts in London, three of which are some distance away. However, the fourth district, Haringey, is adjacent to Friern. It has been decided to demolish the main building of the hospital and to sell off three-quarters of the 30-acre site for development. The remaining quarter will be used to build a central core of psychiatric services for Haringey. This will include an acute admission ward, a variety of small buildings providing sheltered accommodation for chronic patients, and a day activity centre. This is a novel idea which gets round the dismaying problem of finding land in inner London on which to build new facilities. As with the Italian schemes, the long-stay patients on the site could be brought into contact with healthy members of the public who will use the rest of the site, whether it is developed as housing or as a shopping area. These plans result in the public being brought into proximity with the patients, rather than vice versa.

It is very important to discover whether this kind of scheme is beneficial for chronic patients, and one of the main evaluation tasks of TAPS is to compare the Haringey services that develops with that in the Islington health district, which plans to do entirely without the old hospital site.

Prevention of chronicity

The care and treatment of the chronically mentally ill imposes enormous demands on the professional staff involved. For patients discharged after a long stay in a psychiatric hospital, considerable effort is dedicated to creating an artificial social network that will give them the emotional support they need. These patients pose problems of a different order to those of the chronic psychotic individuals in the community catered for by the programs of Stein & Test and of Hoult. The current long-stay population in British psychiatric hospitals consists of three main groups: (a) those who have been left behind by the wave of discharges over the past 35 years because they are so disabled by their illness and/or institutionalism, (b) those who have been discharged in the past but have had to be readmitted because they cannot be contained by existing community facilities, (c) those with a relatively recent onset of an illness which has failed to respond to treatment. Groups (a) and (b) greatly outnumber (c), with the result that the average age of the long-stay, nondemented patients in Friern Hospital is over 60 years.

It would be vastly preferable if therapeutic intervention at the beginning of a career as a psychiatric patient could maintain individuals in their family milieu and prevent the social deterioration that is so often a concomitant of chronicity. Studies of intervention with families of schizophrenic patients have demonstrated that this is possible over a one-year period (Goldstein et al., 1978; Falloon et al., 1982; Leff et al., 1982; Hogarty et al., 1986) and over two years (Falloon et al., 1985; Leff et al., 1985). Whether these innovative treatments benefit patients and their families over a longer period remains to be seen, but the initial findings are very encouraging. They indicate that these methods of working with the families of schizophrenic patients ought to be incorporated into programs such as those initiated by Stein & Test (1980) and Hoult (1986). Equivalent experimental work with other conditions that lead to chronicity might obviate the need for the daunting level of resources that are currently being dedicated to the maintenance of chronically mentally ill patients in the community.

References

Airing, C. D. (1974). The Gheel experience: Eternal spirit of the chainless mind. *Journal of the American Medical Association*, **230**, 998–1001.

Brown, G. W., Birley, J. L. T. & Wing, J. K. (1972). Influence of family life on the course of schizophrenic disorders: A replication. *British Journal of Psychiatry*, **121**, 241–58.

Brown, G. W., Monck, E. M., Carstairs, G. M. & Wing, J. K. (1962). Influence of family life on the course of schizophrenic illness. *British Journal of Preventive and Social Medicine,* **26**, 55–68.

Brown, P. (1985). *The Transfer of Care: Psychiatric Deinstitutionalization and its Aftermath.* Henley-on-Thames: Routledge & Kegan Paul.

Budson, R. D. (1983). Residential Care for the chronically mentally ill. In I. Barofsky & R. D. Budson, eds) *The Chronic Psychiatric Patient in the Community. Principles of Treatment.* New York: Spectrum.

Carpenter, M. D. (1978). Residential placement for the chronic psychiatric patient: a review and evaluation of the literature. *Schizophrenia Bulletin,* **4**, 384–398.

Fagin, L. & Purser, A. (1985). Development of the Waltham Forest local Mental Health Case Register. Unpublished ms.

Fairweather, G. W., Sanders, D. H. & Maynard, H. (1969). *Community life for the Mentally Ill;An Alternative to Institutional Care.* Chicago: Aldine.

Falloon, I. R. H., Boyd, J. L., McGill, C. W., Razani, J., Moss, H. B. & Gilderman, A. (1982). Family management in the prevention of exacerbations of schizophrenia: A controlled study. *New England Journal of Medicine,* **306**, 1437–40.

Falloon, I. R. H., Boyd, J. L., McGill, C. W., Williamson, M., Razani, J., Moss, H. B., Gilderman, A. M. & Simpson, G. M. (1985). Family versus individual management in the prevention of morbidity of schizophrenia: 1. Clinical outcome of a two-year longitudinal study. *Archives of General Psychiatry,* **42**; 887–96.

Faulkner, L. R., Terwilliger, W. B. & Cutler, D. L. (1983). Integrating productive activities into aftercare programs for chronic patients: The Oregon LINC model. In (D. L. Cutler, ed.) *Effective Aftercare for the 1980's: New Directions for Mental Health Services, no. 19,* San Francisco: Jossey-Bass.

Goffman, E. (1961). *Asylums: Essays on the Social Situation of Mental Patients and Other Inmates.* New York: Doubleday.

Goldberg, D. P., Bridges, K., Cooper, W., Hyde, C., Sterling, C. & Wyatt, R. (1985). Douglas House: A new type of hostel ward for chronic psychotic patients. *British Journal of Psychiatry,* **147**, 383–8.

Goldstein, M. J., Judd, L. L., Rodnick, E. H., Alkire, A. A. & Gould, E. (1978). A method for studying social influence and coping patterns within families of disturbed adolescents. *Journal of Nervous and Mental Disease,* **147**, 233–51.

Hogarty, G. E., Anderson, E. M., Reiss, D. J., Kornbluth, S. J., Greenwald, D. P., Javna, C. D. & Madonia, M. J. (1986). Family psychoeducation, social skills training, and maintenance chemotherapy in the aftercare treatment of schizophrenia. 1. One-year effects of a controlled study on relapse and Expressed Emotion. *Archives of General Psychiatry,* **43**, 633–42.

Hoult, J. (1986). Community care of the acutely mentally ill. *British Journal of Psychiatry,* **149**, 137–44.

Johnstone, E. C., Owens, D. G. C., Gold, A., Crow, T. J. & McMillan, J. F. (1981). Institutionalization and the defects of schizophrenia. *British Journal of Psychiatry,* **139**, 195–203.

Johnstone, E. C., Owens, D. G. C., Gold, A., Crow, T. J. & McMillan, J. F. (1984). Schizophrenic patients discharged from hospital – a follow-up study. *British Journal of Psychiatry,* **145,** 586–90.

Leff, J. P., Kuipers, L., Berkowitz, R., Eberlein-Vries, R. & Sturgeon, D. (1982). A controlled trail of social intervention in the families of schizophrenic patients. *British Journal of Psychiatry,* **141,** 121–34.

Leff, J., Kuipers, L., Berkowitz, R. & Sturgeon, D. (1985). A controlled trial of social intervention in the families of schizophrenic patients: two year follow-up. *British Journal of Psychiatry,* **146,** 594–600.

Leff, J. P. & Tress, K. H. (1986). The response of untreated chronic schizophrenics to haloperidol and haloperidol decanoate. *International Clinical Psycho pharmacology,* **1,** Supp. 1 27–10.

Leff, J., Wig, N., Ghosh, A., Bedi, H., Menon, D. K., Kuipers, L., Korten, A., Ernberg, G., Day, R., Sartorius, N. & Jablensky, A. (1987). Influence of relative's Expressed Emotion on the course of schizophrenia in Chandigarh. *British Journal of Psychiatry* **151,** 166–73.

Leff, J. P. & Wing, J. K. (1971). Trial of maintenance therapy in schizophrenia. *British Medical Journal,* iii, 599–604.

Levene, L. S., Donaldson, L. J. & Brandon, S. (1985). How likely is it that a District Health Authority can close its large mental hospitals? *British Journal of Psychiatry,* **147,** 150–3.

Nathan, R. G. & Beigel, A. (1982). Natural support systems: The development of socialization and residential network segments for the chronic patient. (In D. L. Cutler, ed.) *Effective Aftercare for the 1980's: New Directions for Mental Health Services, No. 19.* San Francisco: Jossey-Bass.

NETHRA (1988). North East Thames Regional Health Authority. TAPS evaluation of reprovision for Friern and Claybury Hospitals. Progress Report to the Mental Health Services Evaluation Committee. 1985–8.

Ozarin, L. D. & Levenson, A. I. (1967). The Community Mental Health Centers Program in the U.S.: A new system of mental health care. *Social Psychiatry,* **2,** 145–9.

Stein, L. I. & Test, M. A. (1980). Alternative to mental hospital treatment. I. Conceptual model, treatment program, and clinical evaluation. *Archives of General Psychiatry,* **37,** 392–7.

Sturt, E., Wykes, T. & Creer, C. (1982). Demographic, social and clinical characteristics of the sample. (In J. K. Wing, ed.) Long-term community care: experience in a London Borough. *Psychological Medicine* Monograph Supplement 2.

Vaughn, C. E. & Leff, J. P. (1976). The influence of family and social factors on the course of psychiatric illness: A comparison of schizophrenic and depressed neurotic patients. *British Journal of Psychiatry,* **129,** 125–37.

Warner, R. (1985). *Recovery from Schizophrenia: Psychiatry and Political Economy* London: Routledge and Kegan Paul.

Watt, D. C. & Buglass, D. (1966). The effect of clinical and social factors on the discharge of chronic psychiatric patients. *Social Psychiatry,* **1,** 57–63.

Westermeyer, J. (1980). Psychosis in a peasant society: social outcomes. *American Journal of Psychiatry*, **137**, 1390–4.

Wing, J. K. & Freudenberg, R. K. (1961). The response of severely ill chronic schizophrenic patients to social stimulation. *American Journal of Psychiatry*, **118**, 311–22.

Wing, J. K. & Hailey, A. M. (1972). *Evaluating a Community Psychiatric Service* London: Oxford University Press.

Wykes, T. (1982). A hostel-ward for 'new' long-stay patients: an evaluative study of a 'ward in a house'. In (J. K. Wing, ed.) *Long-term Community Care: Experience in a London Borough. Psychological Medicine.* Supp. 2.

4

Dissemination in New South Wales of the Madison model

John Hoult

'Nothing in the world can take the place of persistence. Talent will not; nothing is more common than unsuccessful men with talent. Genius will not, unrewarded genius is almost a proverb. Education will not; the world is full of educated derelicts. Persistence and determination alone are omnipotent'
Calvin Coolidge, President of USA (1923–9)

In 1979, I undertook a research project in Sydney based on the Stein & Test study of Alternatives to Mental Hospital Care in Madison, Wisconsin. Our project results were similar to Stein & Test's. Four years later in New South Wales, a State Government-commissioned inquiry into services for the psychiatrically ill, influenced by the research results from the project, recommended that Mental Health Services in New South Wales should be restructured using the principles of community care which the research had shown to be effective.

The State Government accepted the Inquiry's report and has made funds available for its implementation, which is now in its fifth year. This article outlines how a research project developed into a system of care.

New South Wales has a population of 5·5 million; its capital city, Sydney, has 3·3 million. For health services, the State is divided into 11 regions which are in turn divided into health areas. Mental health services are predominantly funded by the State Government; it runs the mental hospitals and some community mental health services, and funds general hospitals to provide inpatient psychiatric units and community mental health services. Voluntary organizations do not have an overall significant role as service providers, but there is a large private sector in the main cities which operates independently of the public sector.

Since 1962, the mental hospital census has been declining steadily; it had gone from 9,000 psychiatric residents to fewer than 2,900 in 1983, in spite of the State population increasing by one-third during that time. Community mental health services had been embryonic until 1974, when there was a large injection of funds.

In later years there were cut-backs in community mental health funds. Furthermore, many of the staff tended to focus on the 'worried well', and the chronically mentally ill were often neglected. There was poor liaison between hospital and community staff, and consequent poor continuity of care.

The research project

I had begun working in a community mental health centre in Sydney in 1974. After some years, the deficiencies in the services for the severely mentally ill were increasingly becoming a problem. In 1979, I obtained a Commonwealth Government grant plus State Government funding to undertake a research project which was a replication and extension of the Training in Community Living Project in Madison, Wisconsin, conducted by Stein & Test (1980). Their project used a special team to treat, in the community, a randomized group of patients who had presented for mental hospital admission. The control group was admitted; the experimental group was given intensive treatment and support in the acute phase of their illness, and the team remained responsible for all aspects of follow-up care and treatment in the chronic phase. The results showed that this form of community care produced an outcome which was no worse than, and in some respects superior to, conventional hospital care and follow-up.

Our project ran from 1979–81, and was conducted in suburban Sydney. At the end of the research period, although only the statistics for admission and length of hospital stay were available, it seemed apparent that the project results were going to be favourable, so the Regional Director was keen to establish other such teams in more areas of this region.

Unfortunately, the project completion coincided with a further bout of budgetary contraction; two of the seven project staff were laid off, and for the time being no new teams could be funded. A decision was made to retain the diminished project team as a crisis team incorporated into the local area mental health service.

This was done, and for several years the team functioned successfully in this role. However, budgetary problems were becoming worse, and the only expansion to occur over the next few years was the creation of a small crisis team in an adjoining health area.

In 1983, the results of the research were published in the *Australian and New Zealand Journal of Psychiatry* (Hoult et al., 1983). They were similar to the Stein & Test results, but in addition showed (a) a clear preference by the relatives, and (b) that the experimental treatment was 25 % cheaper. Controversy arose about the project and its results in the correspondence section of the Journal and elsewhere. The project was arousing quite a degree of interest.

The Richmond Inquiry and Report

In the five years prior to 1982, there had been two Health Department committees which examined and reported on mental health services, but no action was taken on their recommendations. The lack of care for the mentally ill had become an increasing theme in the newspapers and television in the late 1970s and early 1980s. Many mentally ill patients were at home imposing a heavy burden on their relatives, who complained of having no support and of being unable to have the patient admitted back to hospital when his behaviour was intolerable. There were recurrent exposés of former patients being neglected, exploited and ill treated in seedy, unregulated boarding houses by unscrupulous owners. And the homeless mentally ill were becoming more of a problem. In 1982, the Minister for Health unexpectedly announced a Public Inquiry into Services for the Psychiatrically Ill and Developmentally Disabled. The majority of the submissions to the Inquiry, both from the general public and from mental health professionals, expressed a great deal of dissatisfaction with existing services; many proposed that services should be set up with a community orientation, espousing the principles of care used in our project. I addressed the Inquiry and spent several hours explaining and advocating for our method of service delivery and answering their questions.

The report of the Inquiry, named after its Chairman, Mr David Richmond, recommended that the highest priority for State Government Mental Health Services should be the community-based care and rehabilitation of the seriously mentally ill. Inpatient and community services for a defined catchment area were to be integrated, all acute psychiatric admission services were to be located in public general hospitals and all admissions to public psychiatric services were to be dependent on prior assessment by a community-based assessment team. The report acknowledged that there would not be unlimited money to set up additional community programmes and services; consequently it recommended that seeding money be given to set up community services which would then have an impact on mental hospital utilization, and the money so saved would be used to set up further community services. Mr Richmond acknowledged that our project had been a model for the new method of service delivery he was recommending.

Quite a deal of uproar ensued upon publication of the report in March 1983. In particular, two unions, the Nurses' Association and the Public Medical Officers' Association, were loud in their condemnation, claiming that the Government wanted to dump patients in the community and sell off the mental hospital land to developers. Not until December 1983 did the Government announce that it would proceed to implement the report, albeit with some concessions to the unions.

The implementation process and the power vacuum

To oversee the implementation of the Report, the Health Department set up a Richmond Implementation Unit in head office. This Unit's function is to call for submissions for programmes for funding from each Health Region, assess the submissions to ensure they conform to the Report's guidelines, allocate money to the Regions and monitor the progress of the new programs. The first year's allocation of money was six million Australian dollars; it was seeding money and was supposed to set up, in each Region, a solid base of services upon which future allocations could build. In subsequent years, the annual allocation of money for staff for new programs was to be repaid to head office from the closure of wards and services in the mental hospitals. The money repaid was then to be used for the next year's allocation for community services.

Formulae were devised to allow for the fact that not all savings in mental hospitals could be materialized at once, especially as the Government promised that no staff would be laid off because of the Richmond Programme. Money was separately provided each year for the purchase of community houses for patients to move into, and for premises to be used for a variety of patient activities. This money for capital expenditure did not have to be repaid.

For ten years there had been no significant focus for Mental health Services in the head office of the Health Department. In 1983, only one psychiatrist was located there. He had no support staff and was severely limited in the time he could give to any one topic. When the Richmond Implementation Unit was set up, for a year or more it included only one person with any clinical mental health experience. It was quickly apparent to several clinicians that a lot of money was going to be spent, but that there was hardly anyone with both a clear understanding of the principles involved in the community-based care of the mentally ill and with relevant clinical experience. There was a great fear that a unique opportunity to improve services for these patients would be lost. Accordingly, a group of us from some of the health regions proposed that we should meet informally with the mental health person on the Richmond Implementation Unit to work out aims and objectives, and to decide on what should be set up. This was a critical step; the group of clinicians who nominated themselves were able to have a major influence on the translation of the broad principles of care enunciated in the report into outlines of practical programs for funding by the Implementation Unit. Equally important, the Richmond Implementation Unit, whom they advised, became the *de facto* Mental Health Directorate of the Health Department because it had support staff. Fortunately this did not present a major problem as the Health Department's senior psychiatrist and the Unit were basically in agreement on most matters.

Implementation – the problems
Because each country has its own unique set of political and administrative structures and functions, the problems encountered will be different. Elsewhere in this volume, Yellowlees and Klerman describe barriers to implementation of

innovative programs. Some of the barriers are painfully familiar to us; Klerman's 'iron triangle' of constituency groups, politicians and Government officials, has impeded our progress too.

Treasury Department

Understandably State Treasury officials were concerned that the program would not fund itself; that the new services would be set up and require recurrent funding, but that administrators and clinicians would then find ways to avoid closing services in the hospitals. These concerns delayed the initial release of money, and each subsequent year almost half the fiscal year elapsed before the final budget for the year was agreed. The fears were warranted, and money was slow in coming out of the mental hospitals.

Other State Government departments

Officials of the Housing Department, which is responsible for public housing in New South Wales, claimed that the Department of Health was about to dump its mentally ill out of the hospitals and into the Housing Department's low-cost houses. For many months they refused to allow any mentally ill people to apply for their houses, whether or not they were hospital patients. Eventually a compromise was reached whereby the Health Department was able to buy 25-year leases from the Housing Department.

Commonwealth Government departments

The care of the mentally ill has always been a State Government responsibility, but in recent times the Commonwealth (i.e. Federal) Government has been partially funding a handful of community-based programmes run by voluntary agencies. With the announcement of the Richmond Report, officials of the Commonwealth accused the State Government of wanting to transfer its costs onto the Commonwealth and refused to fund further projects for the mentally ill.

NSW Health Department administration

Some senior officials had not been too keen to see the mental hospitals decrease in size and number, since they constituted a large part of the Department's work. The Report was considered to be a passing fad, not warranting any effort to drive it along. At a regional level, there were other officials with similar views, and some diverted the Richmond funds into mental health projects contrary to the guidelines.

Mental health professionals

Klerman mentions competing professional ideologies and interprofessional rivalries as a barrier to implementation. This has been a major problem. A considerable number of professionals argued with great conviction against the concept of community care, and disparaged the published reports of successful programs as being the result of charismatic leaders temporarily inspiring a hand-picked team. They opposed the integration of hospital and community services and did not co-operate with others' attempts to achieve this. Interprofessional rivalries were particularly prominent in relation to crisis teams. Psychiatric registrars, used to making decisions about whether or not to admit patients, had disputes with crisis team members who believed they could successfully manage the patients in the community. In a number of hospitals there were bans by doctors on co-operation with crisis teams.

Unions
Right from the start the previously mentioned unions opposed the program – usually not outright, but expressed as a concern either for patients' welfare or for the right of certain professional groups to do particular jobs. In 1985, there were two strikes by nurses in the State mental hospitals, lasting a total of 17 days; in some hospitals the doctors also went on strike for several days. Subsequently, a consultative process was established which worked well in some regions, but elsewhere caused major delays to implementation; this, in turn, affected the amount of money which could be reclaimed from the mental hospitals.

The media
All problems in mental health services were blamed on the Richmond Program. Homelessness, crimes committed by the mentally ill, changes in the interpretation of the Mental Health Act by the legal profession – all were attributed to Richmond, in spite of relatively few patients having been placed, and none of them having been involved in the problems. In fact, the bad publicity came from places where the Richmond Program had not been implemented, but the media did not differentiate.

Implementation – the supports
In spite of all the above problems, the program kept some momentum; it would now be more costly to stop it than to go forward, and whatever the alternative, it would cause greater political unpopularity. Progress at this stage was due to a number of factors.

Clinicians
There were a small but growing group of mental health professionals occupying positions of power in the regions who continued from the original self-appointed advisory group and whose persistence, both at successfully implementing various projects in their regions and in defending the programme from its attackers, ensured its survival.

There has also been an increasing number of mental health professionals working in the new services who have found the experience more satisfying than their previous work and who encourage others to join them; in fact, probably most nonmedical staff who have worked on a well-run new service prefer it to the more traditional service.

Successful projects

These served to keep up the morale of the program's protagonists and to assuage the anxiety of the bureaucracy and the Government that their money might be wasted. Some projects such as crisis teams had a high visibility and their impact in reducing hospital admission rates (sometimes by 50% or more) was instantly recognizable.

Not all the new teams were successful. Some were underfunded and had little impact; some had unclear goals; some lacked adequate leadership. Those that succeeded best owed this to one or two individuals (nurse, social worker, occupational therapist) who became committed to the concepts of the new mode of service delivery and who were able to transmit this to their team. These people were not charismatic (a word often used to denigrate them and the impact they had); they had worked honestly and with commitment in mental hospitals or other parts of the system and brought these qualities with them to the new service. These staff needed nurturing in the early stages, especially those who encountered opposition from the psychiatric profession. Later they formed their own mutual support group which met regularly.

In addition, there were lecture tours of New South Wales by Dr Len Stein and by other mental health professionals from the original Madison project which gave credibility to our own programmes by describing their own successful developments.

Administration

In particular, the program was lucky to have a competent and determined bureaucrat as Manager of the Implementation Unit. Without his persistence with the rest of the bureaucracy, his skilfulness in dealing with politicians and his fierce defence of the program against its attackers, it is likely that the program would not have lasted.

Furthermore, a sufficient number of regional administrators gave support to their committed clinicians, for projects to be initiated and developed in order to demonstrate the potential of the whole program.

At the time of the research project and for some years afterwards, I had been Co-ordinator of Community Mental Health Service for the Lower North Shore Health Area (pop. 150,000) and was responsible for organization of services only within the community component of that Area. When Richmond Implementation was announced, my Regional Director invited me to become the Mental Health Co-ordinator for the Northern Metropolitan Health Region. His reasons were that I had done the research on which a considerable part of the Report was based, and so I should know what programs were required; that doing the research had given me credibility with my peers; and that I was now a persistent advocate for such a program.

The position of Regional Co-ordinator came to have a pivotal role in the Richmond Program. It advised the Richmond Implementation Unit, the Regional Director and the Area Mental Health Service Co-ordinators about what sort of programs to develop and fund. If the Regional Co-ordinator's advice was accepted, then in effect he or she was able to shape the service in the desired way.

Because of the support of the Regional Director and the co-operation and commitment of the psychiatrists who were the Area Service Co-ordinators, the Richmond Program was furthest advanced and had fewest problems in the Northern Metropolitan Region.

Politicians

A program of major change will never succeed without political will. The Minister for Health who commissioned the Richmond Inquiry also had the will to steer the implementation proposal through cabinet in the teeth of strong union opposition. He is an ambitious politician who made his reputation by pushing unpopular causes which he deems necessary. Subsequent Health Ministers maintained the Government's commitment to the Richmond Program, due in part to their own apparent belief that this is the right path to travel, in part to the need for the Government to be seen to be doing something about the problems of the mentally ill and developmentally disabled, and in part to the effectiveness of the advocacy groups mentioned.

Advocacy

Sadly, mental health advocacy groups have not been a powerful lobbying force. On the other hand, in recent years, the relatives of the developmentally disabled have been. On several occasions, when the Richmond Program looked to be under serious threat due to opposition from the unions and from the Government's own fear of the costs, the ability of the developmental disability advocacy groups to lobby politicians certainly saved the program.

They were able to quickly organize a letter-writing campaign to the Minister as well as phone calls and visits to local parliamentarians. Implicit in these actions was their threat to publicly attack the Government. We are now working to build up the mental health advocacy groups to be able to wield such power. We are encouraging them to write to politicians and to visit them; staff have joined their organizations and we have tried to get funds directed to them.

Current position

As the Richmond Program continues into its fifth year, its future looks brighter. Development has been patchy; perhaps five of the eleven regions have done more than set up a few isolated programs. In general, this has reflected the ability, drive and commitment of the Region Co-ordinators, though sometimes even able people have been thwarted by more powerful professionals who are unconvinced by or even opposed to the program.

The aim now is to develop a comprehensive range of community-based services for the mentally ill so that, in metropolitan areas at least, patients can receive all the care they need within their own health area. For the acutely mentally ill, this includes adequate assessment and treatment services based in community mental health centres, a mobile 24-hour crisis team and, for those who do require hospitalization, access to the psychiatric unit in the local general hospital. Only rarely would an acutely mentally ill person need admission to a regional mental hospital for containment. For the chronically mentally ill, a range of services is proposed for each area, much the same as those described by Leff elsewhere in this volume. Each area, for example, would have a range of accommodation facilities, including a 'hospital-hostel' which will be the long-stay facility for its very severely disabled. A variety of work and social programs are proposed as well as family intervention and support programs. Underpinning it all is to be a system of having a 'key-worker' responsible for each patient to ensure he remains in treatment and has his needs adequately addressed. In addition, the Madison concept of having a special Mobile Community Treatment Team to case manage the most noncompliant patients is planned.

There are now nine crisis teams operating in the State, and all five areas of the Northern Metropolitan Health Region have one. A crisis team usually consists of nine staff – typically there are seven nurses, a social worker and a psychologist, though this is not inflexible. Three staff are rostered on the day shift and two on the evening shift, seven days a week. From 11 pm til 8 pm one of the evening shift remains on call, and receives generous penalty rates if called out. The population of the catchment area in the cities varies from 100,000 to 220,000. Where there is more psychiatric disturbance, so there is more staff. A crisis team carries perhaps 30 acute and subacute cases; unfortunately some teams have had to take on a small case-load of disturbed chronic patients because the existing community mental health services are too few (or even unwilling) to care adequately for them. The planned Mobile Community Treatment Teams will be expected to take over the care of these patients.

These teams are very popular with patients and relatives; the latter lobbied the Minister for Health requesting the expeditious establishment of such teams throughout the State. The reasons for their popularity are (a) they are easily contactable and accessible and will come to the house before an episode of illness has progressed too far, (b) the patient knows he is unlikely to be taken off to hospital and so is more willing to co-operate with the team and comply with its treatments, (c) the staff actually spend considerable time talking to the patient and relatives, giving explanations and practical advice, and (d) since the relatives know they can easily get help from the team at any time, they feel secure and are much more willing to continue caring for the patient. As well as crisis teams, day centres providing skills training programmes and social and work programs have been established. Of the patients placed out of the mental hospitals into supported accommodation, almost all have done very well and much prefer the houses to hospital. The first 'hospital-hostel' proved successful and three more have since opened.

Equally important has been the change in staff attitudes and behaviour. There has been an increasing acceptance of the principle that the top priority for Mental Health Services for an area are the severely mentally ill, who are no longer being regarded as unmotivated and unable to be helped. Instead, staff are showing a willingness to be more assertive in their follow-up of these patients, they are using a case management approach and they are supporting relatives much more. In turn, the relatives in a number of areas have formed groups to support local mental health services and are lobbying for increased services.

With the rapid expansion of services, new problems arise. There are too few people of ability and commitment to run the new services; they are swamped with visitors; demands are made on them to train staff for further new services, or to become part-administrators to allow the program to expand to new areas. Their absence sometimes means a good program deteriorates. There is no good mechanism to ensure quality control, and so quality is very much dependent on the calibre of the person running the programme. Ideally, there would be a system of benevolent supervision, where an experienced clinician would regularly assess the quality of care and the progress of the service, and would assist in overcoming obstacles. The problems of establishing and of expanding the services in difficult financial times means that there is no money to employ anyone in this job; usually a tragedy or a scandal is necessary before this position gets funded. A scheme is being proposed whereby a standard form of service evaluation can be used, thus enabling comparisons to be made. However, its use is voluntary. Accreditation is another means of quality assurance, but it too has its problems and is a long way off.

In early 1987 the Regional Director of the Southern Metropolitan Region, where the Richmond Program had struck considerable obstacles, asked me to transfer to that region to help overcome the obstacles and speed up implementation of the programme. The unions in the two mental hospitals there had been at the forefront of opposition to the program, to the extent that they had blocked transfers of patients and closure of wards, thereby preventing the release of funds from the hospitals to drive the next stage of the program. In addition, the region did not have a psychiatrist who was a champion of the Richmond Program; this meant that negotiations with the health areas were hampered because the psychiatrists in the areas really prefer to negotiate with a psychiatrist.

I believe the Southern Metropolitan Region is the key region in New South Wales for this program. It contains the Skid Row district of Sydney, and several of the health areas of the region score highest in indices of poverty and social disorganisation. If the Richmond Program can work effectively in this region, it can work anywhere in urban Australia. Furthermore, the two medical schools in Sydney are both located in the Southern Metropolitan Region, together with the majority of the teaching hospitals; if they come to accept and to actively support the programme, it will become the standard way of service delivery.

Principles for change agents

In attempting to distil out of our particular experience some general principles to help others who might be tempted to try to disseminate their own innovate mental . health program, I am aware that the path is already trodden. The principles ennunciated by Fairweather *et al.* (1974) help guide me, and now Backer *et al.* (1986) have summarized recent knowledge. I have little to add that is new; I can only confirm or change the emphasis. Nevertheless, the principles need reiterating, and I shall do so in my own words.

Clear goals

We knew right from the beginning – and we still know – what we wanted to achieve. There have been adjustments along the way, in the light of our own experience or information from the literature, but the main goal has remained firm. There has also been a fixed commitment to the severely mentally ill as our target group.

Persistence

Of all the components, this is the most important. It cannot be stressed too much. The necessity to keep going in the face of frustrations, delays, and opposition is vital. Fairweather *et al.*, (1974, p. 195) put it truly: 'perseverance may not pay off, but change can not happen without it'. The number of persistent champions of the program has grown over the years, but most importantly, many of the original champions are still involved. Successful innovative programs sometimes do not progress beyond the demonstration stage because the innovators move on and do not commit themselves to the development phase. In New South Wales, half the staff of the original project are still involved in this sort of work (so much for 'burn-out').

Exploiting opportunities

Unique events or circumstances occur during the course of disseminating any program; they need to be taken advantage of in order to progress towards the goal. In our case, several opportunities stand out.

The perceived need for change: There had been increasing dissatisfaction throughout New South Wales with the nonsystem of care that existed prior to 1983. Though they might not all agree with the new proposals, everyone was ready for change and wanting change.

Filling the power vacuum: The absence of a powerful clinician (or group of clinicians) responsible for the direction of mental health services meant that new proposals did not threaten a pre-existing ideology or power structure. The clinicians committed to the new proposals, who became the self-appointed and unofficial advisers to the Richmond Implementation Unit, in effect came to wield considerable power within the organization, for the want of any alternative. Once the power vacuum was filled, the relatively centralized nature of the Health Department meant that it was much easier to implement the new principles of care statewide than it would have been in a more decentralized and locally autonomous organization.

Control of resources allocation: Virtually the only new money coming into mental health services in the past five years has been Richmond Implementation money. This has given a lot of power to the Richmond Implementation Unit and to Regional Mental Health Co-ordinators to shape services. All Area Mental Health Services want new resources, so they are prepared to negotiate and to accept Richmond guidelines to obtain them. Not only does the new program have to conform to the Richmond guidelines, but the opportunity is then taken to bring existing services more into line with the general Richmond direction so that the new services will not be isolated.

Citizen advocacy

Although the advocacy groups for the developmentally disabled were not especially concerned with the mentally ill, their pressure on the Government at one crucial stage saved the programme. Their constant pressure on the Department of Health and the Government has helped to maintain momentum of the whole program, not just the section for the developmentally disabled. Mental health services have been pulled along in their wake.

Credibility

We have constantly been concerned to ensure our credibility. Even though Stein and Test's research was methodologically sound and had been widely acclaimed (and hence credible) it was still attacked as being only relevant for the USA and for a city like Madison. Our research project had similar methodology to Stein &

Test's and had similar results. It demonstrated clearly that their principles were valid for the metropolitan areas of Australia.

The replication impressed our administrators, our clinicians and finally the Richmond Inquiry. It made refutation of criticisms a great deal easier; in debate it is a powerful weapon to be able to point to one's own research evidence and then ask the opposition where is theirs. Publication of our own results in local and international journals (Reynolds & Hoult, 1984) and invitations to give lectures overseas (Hoult, 1986) further implied scientific acceptance of the research.

The credibility was maintained as the program progressed.

Several of the crisis teams set up with Richmond funds quickly had a significant impact. Admission rates from their catchment areas fell by 50% or more, and wards were left with empty beds. This impact was brought to the attention of senior bureaucrats and the Minister for Health, and together with the enthusiastic response of the relatives to these teams, had a powerful effect in convincing them of the correctness of the new directions. It also helped refute those critics within the health professions who claimed the successful project results were due to the unique motivation of a special research team and would not be replicated in routine practice. Lecture tours of New South Wales by Dr Len Stein and later by other health professionals from the Madison Service also helped to shift attitudes in our direction.

Personal contact

Backer *et al.* (1986), in their review of the characteristics of effective dissemination of innovative psychosocial interventions, mention that this is almost always an essential component. I wholeheartedly agree. Face-to-face contact has been vital to get others to accept the innovation and support it and act on it. This applies both up the line in the bureaucratic organisation, and with peers.

Regarding the bureaucracy, often I have heard colleagues bemoaning the failure of their written submissions and proposals to gain acceptance. Those written submissions and proposals which are left to find their own way in the world solely on their merits do not go far. Success depends on persistent but appropriate lobbying of the bureaucrat who has the power to make the desired decision or who can influence on your behalf the decision-maker. People have to be coaxed, cajoled, convinced about the value of the new proposal, just as a salesman has to sell a product. Personal contact works the other way, too; it means they are much more likely to inform you about potential opportunities or problems, so that you can take appropriate and timely action.

With regard to peers, the principle still holds. For example, the most successful crisis teams have been set up by the staff of the original project team, or by a newcomer who has developed a strong link with one of the original team; and who became committed to the principles. The least successful teams have had the least contact. Personal contact also allows the program champion in a new team, or a team which is experiencing problems, to turn easily to the person who introduced the new ideas to get advice, guidance and support. This has helped sustain teams through quite frustrating and difficult periods where little except a holding operation was being achieved. Our new teams also have a system of regular meetings or forums where they exchange information and give mutual support; these have proved very valuable.

Organizational support

This enabled the various stages to be successfully traversed. Initially, it was the Regional Director and his staff who helped to get the funding for the research project, and who enabled the project to survive during the first two years following the completion of the research. (In retrospect, this was the most difficult and frustrating period of the whole eight years.) Once the Inquiry was announced, the organizational support needed to be moved to a higher level; it became important to secure the support of officials within the central administration of the Health Department. Then, when the principles of care in the research became policy, it was necessary to ensure that the Department's top administration and the Government were supportive and remained so.

Fairweather *et al.* (1974) state that they found there was a limited role of formal authority *vis-à-vis* change. Given the nature and extent of the changes we wanted to make, and the power structures within the New South Wales Health Department, I would disagree with those authors; I consider our progress would have been a great deal slower – perhaps by a decade or more – without organizational support. The critical element for us was that it gave us control of the new money to be allocated.

Limiting opposition

We have tried to avoid fighting on too many fronts at once. A program such as ours which challenges the accepted way of doing things must attract opposition from those who feel their jobs, their power or their ideology are threatened. The Government has made concessions to the nursing unions about mental hospital staff having priority for jobs in the new services. We have stressed to psychiatrists and registrars that their 'ultimate responsibility' is not challenged in the new services. These actions help to constrain the debate to areas of ideology and data, and here the latter is in our favour.

Adaptability

Backer *et al.* (1986) comment on the controversy on this point. Although we tried to ensure conformity by having the new services in an area undergo training with the best of the established services, ultimately the local management have been free to make their own adaptations. Those services which varied the most from the original model were also those which had leaders least committed to the model, and the latter factor seemed more important in accounting for poor performance.

Later developments

In mid-1987, following a number of unexplained deaths in state mental hospitals, the Minister for Health set up a Ministerial Advisory Committee to investigate standards of care in them. The committee included three psychiatrists; namely a Professor of psychiatry, the senior psychiatrist of the Health Department, and probably the most respected senior private psychiatrist in Sydney. The recommendations of the Committee were released in September. The first recommendation was that all mental hospitals should close within five years. Community-based residential and support services were to be provided before any closures occurred.

The Minister announced that only five mental hospitals would close within the next five years; three would remain. He simultaneously announced that the Government would give an additional 200 million Australian dollars to the mental health system over the next eight years to set up further crisis teams, community support teams, day centres, work programmes and sheltered accommodation. Special teams and facilities were to be set up for the homeless mentally ill, and small 16-bed units in the Community were to be established for the confused and disturbed elderly. The Minister said New South Wales would have a comprehensive network of services for the mentally ill unparalleled in the world. However, most of the funding for the new services was to come from the closure of the hospitals.

The Ministerial announcement started up the opposition again. The unions embarked on a vigorous media campaign against the new initiatives, and banned the transfer of patients from mental hospitals to any new community facility. In Parliament, the Opposition attacked the Government over its new plans and promised the unions to keep the mental hospitals open if they won the next election. After the usual delay, the Government released funding to recruit staff for the first wave of new services. Top priority was given to the inner city area where the homeless mentally ill congregate, but many other services were planned for 1988. However, in March 1988 the Government went early to the polls, and lost.

The new Government immediately ceased all recruitment; only the inner city service beat the cut-off. Another Ministerial Committee was appointed to come up with yet another plan. The unions were heavily represented on this Committee, whereas no one with any community experience was a member. The Committee did not call for any submissions. Its Report, in December 1988, advised the Government to keep all of the State's mental hospitals and to spend $80 million to refurbish and rebuild wards. However, they did not go so far as to recommend increasing the capacity or the staffing of the hospitals, they did not propose reductions in any existing community mental health services and they even recommended the establishment of further crisis teams and other community services, albeit at a slower rate, with a reduced staffing level and without sufficient back-up supports such as residentials and intensive support teams. The new Government accepted the Committee's Report and said it would implement it.

In its Report, the Committee acknowledged that at least 95% of patients with severe mental illness now reside outside the mental hospitals, and that the existing mental hospital population will probably decline further. In spite of this, the major thrust of their plan is the mental hospitals; 85% of public mental health money will still be devoted to 5% of the patients. Patients outside hospital will still lead impoverished lives, still cause suffering to their relatives, and still relapse far too frequently because there are insufficient services that help them. And while the newly established service in the inner city has ensured that the homeless mentally ill are now taking medication and no longer causing disturbances in the shelters, other patients in suburbs where there are inadequate services are relapsing, becoming homeless and drifting into the shelters. Moreover, although the new service is now placing improved homeless patients into priority housing in the suburbs, those without support will soon relapse and return to homelessness. The Committee has not grasped that only when all areas have adequate numbers of community mental health staff, providing a comprehensive range of services targeted at the severely mentally ill, together with an assertive case manager system, only then will the problems of the mentally ill begin to be resolved.

The good news was that clinicians and bureaucrats from the neighbouring state of Victoria had come to New South Wales in 1987 to observe our new developments. In 1988, they commenced the first of their new services based on the model we had been developing, and more were planned for 1989. Again, a similar positive response from patients and relatives was noted, and hospital admissions were down.

In New South Wales we must wait until the new Government learns that its preoccupation with the hospitals is not going to resolve the problems of the mentally ill. I doubt this will take more than a couple of years, then we must take up the struggle again, Calvin Coolidge was right – perseverance is all.

Conclusion

Although it has been gratifying to see the improvements in service delivery which have occurred, and to note the improved attitudes of patients, relatives and staff, the task has been long and becomes increasingly complex. The initial research project was mainly a clinical task. To set it on the road to becoming a Statewide system of care has meant that clinicians have had to become involved on administrative, industrial, economic and political fronts, as well as maintaining the clinical one. These fronts are foreign to clinicians, but they must be engaged if change is to occur. Furthermore, a range of allies and supporters has had to be sought, won over and encouraged; one person alone cannot change everything. Most of all, there is need for persistence in the face of the early setbacks and inertia that will inevitably occur. Systems can change. In mental health it is important that they do. I hope our effort will encourage and help others.

References

Backer, T. E., Liberman, R. P. & Kuehnel, T. G. (1986). Dissemination and Adoption of Innovative Psychosocial Interventions *Journal of Consultative and Clinical Psychology*, **54**, 111–18,

Fairweather, G. W., Sanders, D. H. & Tornatzky, L. G. (1974). *Creating Change in Mental Health Organisations*. New York: Pergamon Press.

Hoult, J. (1986). Community Care of the Acutely Mentally Ill. *British Journal of Psychiatry*, **149**, 137–44.

Hoult, J., Reynolds, I., Charbonneau-Powis, M., Weekes, P. & Briggs, J. (1983). Psychiatric Hospital Versus Community Treatment: The Results of Randomised Trial. *Australian and New Zealand Journal of Psychiatry* **17**, 160–7.

Reynolds, I. & Hoult, J. (1984). The Relatives of the Mentally Ill: A Comparative Trial of Community Oriented and Hospital Oriented Care. *Journal of Nervous and Mental Disease*, **172**, 480–9.

Stein, L. I. & Test, M. A. (1980). Alternative to Mental Hospital Treatment: 1. Conceptual Model, Treatment Program and Clinical Evaluation. *Archives of General Psychiatry*, **37**, 392–7.

Section B: Primary care

Editors' commentary

A transforming new perspective in mental health care comes from the new knowledge we have gained about where most clinical problems are and what their nature is. Far more mental health problems are present in primary care than in any other setting. The huge scale of this psychiatric ill health, detailed in this section by Katon from the United States and Paykel from the United Kingdom, has only become widely appreciated in recent years. This unveiling of mental morbidity in the late twentieth century parallels the disclosure from public health studies a century earlier of the prevalence of physical illness in Europe and North America.

What are these mental health problems in primary care? The diagnostic categories used by psychiatrists largely evolved in hospital samples and are less easy to apply in primary care. Most sufferers are the 'ambulant wounded' with anxious-depressive symptoms, often with problems in living. They lack a reliable nosology. The label of 'minor' psychiatric illness can mislead. It obscures the fact that many cases are not of brief mild adjustment reactions that soon remit. Often the problem is chronic over many years and anxiety disorders in the community are commonly handicapped socially (Weissman, 1989). Some cases with severe obsessive-compulsive disorders are at least as chronically handicapped as are chronic schizophrenics. Furthermore, as 'community care' grows, so chronic psychotics become more obvious in the case-loads of primary carers.

Much psychiatric morbidity goes unrecognized, as Katon and Paykel emphasize. Neither patients nor carers always give such problems or their management a mental health label. We can speak prose all our lives without knowing it, and in care delivery the label need not be crucial to giving appropriate treatment. Yet

58

recognizing problems for what they are can sharpen awareness of them, refine their management, and ultimately lead to better understanding and prevention. Many patients have comorbidity of both physical and psychiatric difficulties, the somatic symptoms distracting the primary carer from mental health aspects of the problem which are then neglected.

Although it is desirable that primary care physicians should become better able to spot such problems, we lack a reliable technology to help them do so. Education is not always productive. After two years' work with a psychiatrist and a nurse therapist, general practitioners still missed cases of anxiety disorder suitable for behavioural treatment (Marks, 1985).

Given that most mental health troubles are seen for the first time by nonspecialist primary carers, if the problems are spotted how can they be helped by the nonspecialist? It seems most economic and desirable to treat them in the primary care setting, given the frequent reluctance of sufferers to incur a potential stigma from attending a psychiatric facility. Only the hardest cases need secondary or tertiary referral.

Much of the anxiety/depression and problems in living seen in primary care are treated by brief counselling/psychotherapy and/or medication. Paykel describes an innovative research finding that brief counselling reduced psychotropic drug use. Other work found that depressives in primary care benefit from adequate doses of an antidepressant drug but often get either none at all or too little. Primary care physicians need education about this.

Another innovation mentioned here is the successful delivery of primary mental health care by new personnel moving into primary care. Nurses and social workers have produced encouraging improvement in marital problems, depression and anxiety disorders, using casework counselling and behavioural methods. Psychologists and psychiatrists are working increasingly in primary care as well as in hospital settings.

This section touches on fiscal barriers to improving primary mental health care. Funding rules may obstruct the optimum deployment of personnel. If a new care pattern by care authority A makes great savings for the community overall (care authorities B–Z) but costs A something, then that innovation is unwelcome to A unless A is recompensed. A potential solution is suggested by the current nine-cities initiative for the seriously mentally ill (SMI) from the Robert Wood Johnson Foundation (RWJ); RWJ gives incentive for all authorities responsible for some aspect of mental health care for the SMI in a city to get together as a single co-ordinated agency within which funds can be moved as needed.

References

Marks, I. M. (1985). Psychiatric nurse therapy in primary care: A controlled study. Book in *Research Series of Royal College of Nursing*, Henrietta Street, London, WC2.

Weissman, M. (1989). Paper to Regional Conference on Nonpsychotic Disorders, Jerusalem. April.

5

Implications for care delivery of mental illness in primary care

Wayne Katon

This chapter will focus on four major points:

1. Of patients with mental illness, 50 to 60% in the United States are treated exclusively in primary care;
2. Primary care physicians have been found in many studies to frequently overlook mental illness;
3. Somatization (the presentation of psychosocial distress in a somatic idiom and health care seeking behaviour) is the major cause of infrequent recognition of mental illness by medical physicians;
4. There is a high cost to society from unrecognized and untreated mental illness due to the:
    (a) High medical use by somatizing patients with psychosocial problems and the resulting, frequently costly and dangerous high technology medical testing they are exposed to.
    (b) Chronic illness behaviour that these patients have with job absenteeism and chronic disability payments often ensuing.
    (c) Resulting family disfunction that frequently leads to somatic complaints and high medical use by other family members.

Numerous studies have demonstrated that 30 to 50% of patients in primary care use medical care secondary to psychosocial stress and problems (Stoeckle et al., 1964; Culpan & Davies, 1960). Of primary care patients 25 to 33% meet research criteria for psychiatric illness (Hoeper et al., 1979). Approximately 50% of primary care visits are secondary to stress and 50 to 60% of United States patients with mental illness are treated exclusively in primary care (Regier et al., 1978, 1984).

Over six months, 70% of patients with mental illness were seen in primary care, whereas only 20% visited a mental health professional (Regier *et al.*, 1984).

In a large study of over 500,000 patients visiting 188 primary care physicians in Virginia, anxiety and depression made up 87% of the psychiatric illnesses seen (Marsland *et al.*, 1976). The more severe illnesses such as schizophrenia, manic-depressive illness and dementia are preferentially referred to the mental health sector of care. Of primary care patients 27% met RDC for mental illness, with depression occurring in 6% of patients (Hoeper *et al.*, 1979). That makes depression the most common clinical problem seen in primary care, with hypertension next at 5·7% of the population.

Primary care patients frequently have comorbidity – both chronic medical illness and psychiatric illness. The most frequent precipitant of depression in an elderly population was acute physical illness in the patient or spouse (Murphy, 1982). Psychiatric illness frequently worsens the course of chronic medical illness in adversely affecting self-monitoring and maintenance care (taking medication, staying on a diet, exercising), and it amplifies complaints (Surridge *et al.*, 1984).

Not only is mental illness exceedingly common in primary care patients, but those with mental illness use two to three times as much medical care as patients without medical illness (for review, see Hankin & Oktay 1979). The study by Weissman and colleagues (1981) is typical in finding a high frequency of mental illness in the community, high use of medical care by these patients and the frequent lack of recognition of the mental illness by physicians. In a large epidemiological study of the New Haven community (Weissman *et al.*, 1981) 4·3% of people in the community who had a structured interview met Research Diagnostic Criteria (Spitzer *et al.*, 1982) for major depression. Two-thirds of these patients were receiving no medical care for this serious mental illness and 65% of these patients with undiagnosed mental illness made six or more visits to their primary care physicians over one-year – more visits than from patients without major depression. Over 50% of these patients with major depression were prescribed a sedative-hypnotic (probably for nonspecific somatic complaints like tension or insomnia) whereas only 17% had tricyclic antidepressants.

Why is the recognition rate of mental illness by primary care physicians so low? Paykel (1990–Chap. 6, this volume) has suggested two reasons based on physician practices. First, primary care physicians in the United Kingdom on average spend 7·5 minutes per patient compared to the half to one hour of psychiatrists, and primary care physicians tend to focus on the patient's chief complaint, which is usually somatic. Second, in the United States there is a financial disincentive to spending time with patients especially when compared to reimbursement for procedures. In the United Kingdom, most physicians are salaried within the National Health Service and there is no financial incentive to refer for procedures or tests.

Other studies suggest that a major patient-determined reason for the lack of diagnosis of mental illness is somatization. The National Ambulatory Medical Care survey found that 70% of patients with a psychiatric illness present with a somatic complaint (Shurman *et al.*, 1985). Goldberg (1979) also found both in the United States and the United Kingdom that over 50% of patients with anxiety and depression present to their primary care physician with a somatic complaint. The most convincing study to show how somatization causes physicians to overlook mental illness (Bridges & Goldberg, 1985) was of 497 new inceptions of illness (new complaints that the patient had not talked to a physician about for one year). Before their consultation with their physician, patients had a structured psychiatric interview and were asked why they consulted their physician. Of the patients, 54% had an entirely physical illness, 13% had an adjustment reaction and 33% met DSM-III criteria for one or more psychiatric illnesses (Bridges & Goldberg, 1985). Two-thirds of the patients with psychiatric illness also had one or more chronic physical illnesses. Of the 33% of patients with psychiatric illness, 32% presented with a somatic complaint they believed was due to a medical illness but none was found, 27% complained about chronic physical illness, 17% had psychological symptoms and 24% presented with 'facultative somatization' (they told the research team of their psychiatric illness, but told their physician only of their somatic, not psychological, symptoms).

Bridges & Goldberg (1985) then studied the recognition of mental illness by primary care physicians. Of the patients who presented psychological symptoms 94% were recognized as having these, 73% of patients with mental illness were recognized when their psychiatric illness was secondary to a physical one, 23% of patients with mental illness were recognized when their psychiatric illness was unrelated to a physical one but both were present, and only 50% of these patients were recognized as having psychiatric illness when somatization occurred. The presentation of somatic symptoms and/or chronic medical illness seemed to distract the primary care physician from recognizing the patients' psychological and social state.

Freeling *et al.* (1985) found that primary care patients with unrecognized depression, compared to patients recognized as depressed by their family physician, had:

1. less overt depressed mood and appearance.
2. less insight about their psychological condition.
3. been depressed longer.
4. been more likely to have suffered their depression secondary to a physical illness.

The purpose of this paper was to describe the main obstacles and barriers to improved mental health care within the primary care system and to suggest strategies to overcome these barriers. The above data make it apparent that any innovation in the care and treatment of mental disorder in the primary care system must take into account the following factors:

1. Many patients perceive their mental illness as entirely physical or somatopsychic (secondary to medical illness).

2. Many primary care patients have co-morbidity – mental plus physical illness – and it is often difficult for them and their physicians to distinguish symptoms of mental illness from those of physical illness.

3. Many patients are quite defensive about having a mental illness. Tyrer (1984) found that about 20% of patients who were treated by a psychiatrist working in a primary care practice said they would not have attended a separate psychiatric facility had they been sent there.

4. Often somatizers' illness behaviour is reinforced by second gains (beneficial changes in one's family and vocational system or larger social support system) (Katon et al., 1981).

5. Many patients refuse referral to mental health practitioners. Thus, 74% of physicians felt that patient resistance to mental health referral was a significant obstacle to effective treatment (Orlean et al., 1985).

6. The United States third-party reimbursement schedules that pay preferentially for procedures and penalize time spent with patients significantly affect the ability of physicians to recognize mental illness. In Great Britain the brief time (mean of 7·7 minutes) that primary care physicians spend with patients impedes their ability to accurately diagnose mental illness.

Paykel (1990, this volume, chapter 6), reviewed the literature on the many studies that have looked at the cost-effectiveness of differing schemes of treatment of mental illness in primary care. In these days of continual assault on the high cost of medical care by government, third party payers and the public, evidence is essential that it is cost-effective to diagnose and treat patients with mental illness who present to primary care physicians.

Several methodological problems with the studies Paykel (1990, this volume, chapter 6), reviewed make it unlikely that cost-effectiveness would be proved. First, most of the studies either screen patients for mental illness and then helped those they found, by psychotherapy or pharmacotherapy, or they simply looked at medical records of patients who had had psychotherapy (Mumford et al., 1984). The problem with both these approaches is that although patients with mental illness on average use more medical care, this may not be true of all patients with mental illness. Probably those who use the most medical care view their mental illness as a physical one. Yet the patients chosen for the cost-offset psychotherapy studies are by definition 'psychologizers' who are probably not high users of medical care. Thus the 'somatizers' of psychosocial distress who are probably the highest users of health care are not included in these cost-offset studies. In our own studies patients with chronic pain used a tremendous amount of medical resources. Patients with chronic back, pelvic, and chest pain had very high rates of psychiatric illness that often preceded the onset of pain (Katon *et al.*, 1985, Walker *et al.*, 1982).

A second point is that many studies included patients with minor mental illness which often resolves without treatment (Johnstone & Goldberg, 1976). In two studies of patients with depression in primary care, about half the patients were no longer depressed six months later (Hankin & Locke, 1979; Mann *et al.*, 1981).

A third point is that most studies have not adequately described or structured the psychological intervention, beyond calling it long- or short-term psycho-therapy. This therapy most likely varied from practitioner to practitioner and was probably short-term (two to eight visits) having nonspecific effects. An exception here is the work of Marks (1985 *a, b*) in Great Britain in primary care where specific carefully defined short-term behavioural treatments led to significantly more improvement than in controls who had non-behavioural treatment from their family doctor.

There are several methodological strategies that would enhance the researchers' ability to study those patients who are both most difficult for physicians – patients who somatize – and most likely to increase the cost of medical care due to frequent visits and unnecessary medical evaluations (laboratory exams, X-rays, CAT scans). Bridges & Goldberg's (1985) studies and our own from the University of Washington suggest that the most difficult of these patients are those with co-morbidity – both psychiatric and chronic medical illness. The physician's anxiety that they may miss an exacerbation of the patient's medical problem distracts from the search for psychosocial cures to symptoms.

One strategy would be to study treatment outcome in consistently high users of medical care who also have a mental disorder over one to two years or more. Patients with heterogeneous symptoms could have specific (medication/ psychotherapy, behavioural treatment aimed at illness behaviour) or nonspecific interventions (consultation–liaison psychiatrist supervision of primary care practitioners).

Another strategy would be to study the effect of a specific treatment in consistently high users who have one symptom (chest pain, back pain, headache) and a negative organic workup, or one chronic illness (diabetes) with coexistent major depression.

Such designs using clearly defined specific treatment or a mode of treatment (consultation–liaison supervision of family physician) and a cost–benefit analysis with an economic consultant would tell us more about the value of psychological interventions with difficulty and costly somatizers.

Future studies could address the following questions.

1. Does improved accuracy of diagnosis and early detection of mental disorder decrease patient's symptoms, increase family adaptation, and reduce medical costs and absenteeism and job disability? A liaison psychiatrist could supervise primary care physicians in interview and treatment of high users with both heterogeneous and homogeneous somatic symptoms.

2. Does drug treatment of somatizers with major depression and panic disorder decrease their symptoms, utilization and medical costs? Again, a liaison psychiatrist/primary care physician team would optimally test these interventions in a primary care clinic.

3. Do short-term interpersonal, cognitive-behavioural, behavioural or marital psychotherapy treatments decrease utilization, medical and psychological symptoms and illness behaviour? Here psychiatric nurses or social workers who work within the primary care clinic could test a specific type of psychotherapy on disorders such as:
   (a) major depression.
   (b) panic disorder.
   (c) marital disfunction and/or sexual disfunction.
   (d) poor compliance with medical treatment of specific illnesses such as hypertension or diabetes.

Conclusion

Many patients with mental illness are seen exclusively within the primary care system. They use a great deal of medical resources, especially in the United States where somatizers often have high technology, expensive and often invasive tests. The primary care clinic is a nonstigmatizing system in which to develop treatment interventions for mental illness, and patients often prefer it to the mental health system. Research strategies are outlined to test mental health treatment interventions in high utilizing primary care patients.

References

Bridges, K. W. & Goldberg, D. P. (1985). Somatic presentation of DSM-III psychiatric disorders in primary care. *Journal of Psychosomatic Research*, **29**, 563–9.

Culpan, R. & Davies, B. (1960). Psychiatric illness at a medical and surgical outpatient clinic. *Comparative Psychiatry*, **1**, 228–35.

Freeling, P., Rao, B. M., Paykel, E. S., Sireling, L. I. & Burton, R. H. (1985). Unrecognized depression in general practice. *British Medical Journal* **290**, 1880–3.

Goldberg, D. (1979). Detection and assessment of emotional disorders in a primary care setting. *International Journal of Mental Health*, **8**, 30–48.

Hankin, J. & Locke, B. Z. (1982). The persistence of depression symptomatology in prepaid group practice enrollees: An exploratory study. *American Journal of Public Health*, **72**, 1000–9.

Hankin, J. & Oktay, J. S. (1979). Mental disorder and primary medical care: An analytic review of the literature. In *National Institute of Mental Health* (Rockville, MD): Series D, No. 7, DHEW Publication No. (ADM) 78–661. Government Printing Office.

Hoeper, E. W., Nyczi, G. P., Cleary, P. D., Regier, D. & Goldberg, I. (1979). Estimated prevalence of RDC mental disorder in Primary Care. *International Journal of Mental Health*, **8**, 6–15.

Johnstone, A. & Goldberg, D. (1976). Psychiatric screening in general practice: A controlled trial. *Lancet*, **1**, 605–8.

Katon, W., Egan, K. & Miller, D. (1985). Chronic pain: Lifetime psychiatric diagnoses and family history. *American Journal of Psychiatry*, **142**, 1156–60.

Katon, W., Hall, M. P., Russo, J., Cormier, L., Hollifield, M. & Beitman, B. (1988). Chest Pain: The Relationship of psychiatric illness to coronary arteriography results. *American Journal of Medicine*, **84**, 1–9.

Katon, W., Kleinman, A. & Rosen, G. (1981). Depression and somatization: A review. Part II. *American Journal of Medicine*, **72**, 241–247.

Mann, A. H., Jenkins, R. & Belsey, E. (1981). The twelve-month outcome of patients with neurotic illness in general practice. *Psyclinological Medicine*, **11**, 535–50.

Marks, I. M. (1985 a). Controlled trial of psychiatric nurse therapists in primary care. *British Medical Journal*, **290**, 1181–4.

Marks, I. M. (1985 b), *Psychiatric nurse therapists in primary care*. Royal College of Nursing, London.

Marsland, D. W., Wood, M. & Mayo, F. (1976). A data bank for patient care, curriculum and research in family practice: 526,196 patient problems. *Journal of Family Practice*, **3**, 25.

Mumford, E., Schlesinger, H. J., Glass, G. V., Patrick, C. & Cuerdon, T. (1984). A new look at evidence about reduced cost of medical utilization following mental health treatment. *American Journal of Psychiatry*, **141**, 1145–58.

Murphy, F. (1982). Social origins of depression in old age. *British Journal of Psychiatry*, **141**, 135–42.

Orlean, C. T., George, L. K., Houpt, J. L. & Brodie (1985). How primary care physicians treat psychiatric disorders. A national survey of family practitioners. *American Journal of Psychiatry*, **142**, 52–7.

Regier, D. A., Goldberg, I. D., Taube, C. A. (1978). The *de facto* U.S. mental health services system. *Archives in General Psychiatry*, **35**, 685.

Regier, D. A., Myers, J. K., Kramer, M., Robins, L. N., Blazer, D. G., Hough, R. L., Eaton, W. W. & Locke, B. Z. (1984). The NIMH Epidemiologic Catchment

Area (ECA) Program: Historical context major objectives, and study population characteristics. *Archives in General Psychiatry*, **41**, 934–41.

Shurman, R. A., Kramer, P. D. & Mitchell, J. B. (1985). The hidden mental health network: Treatment of mental illness by nonpsychiatrist physicians. *Archives in General Psychiatry*, **42**, 89–94.

Spitzer, R. L., Endicott, J. & Robins, E. (1982). Research Diagnostic Criteria– Rationale and Reliability. *Archives in General Psychiatry*, **35**, 773–82.

Stoeckle, J. D., Zola, J. K. & Davidson, G. E. (1964). The quantity and significance of psychological distress in medical patients. *Journal of Chronic Diseases*, **17**, 959.

Surridge, D. H. C., Williams, R., Erdahl, D. L., Lawson, J. S. (1984). Psychiatric aspects of diabetes mellitus. *British Journal of Psychiatry*, **145**, 269–76.

Tyrer, P. (1984). Psychiatric clinics in general practice: An extension of community care. *British Journal of Psychiatry*, **145**, 9–14.

Walker, E., Katon, W., Harrop-Griffiths, J., Russo, J. & Hickok, L. (1988). Chronic pelvic pain: The relationship to psychiatric diagnoses and childhood sexual abuse. *American Journal of Psychiatry*, **145**, 75–80.

Weissman, M. M., Myers, J. K., Thompson, W. D. (1981). Depression and its treatment in a U.S. urban community 1975–1976. *Archives in General Psychiatry*, **38**, 417–21.

6

Innovations in mental health care in the primary care system

Eugene Paykel

Characteristics of health care and disorder in primary care

It is appropriate that a contributor from the United Kingdom should deal with mental health care in primary care, since, as is well known, the British National Health Service is strongly rooted in primary care. In theory, every person in the country is registered with a general practitioner and has continuity of comprehensive care with that doctor, who knows his history well. Consultation with the GP is the first step in care for psychiatric disorder, with the pathway to specialist care being by secondary referral, and only in a minority of cases. The average GP has about 2,100 patients on his list.

In practice of course there are gaps and departures from the ideal in the system. For instance, some persons, particularly the deprived and rootless, do not register with a GP; some GPs have little acquaintance with their patients and knowledge of the person and the family context is only acquired slowly. Nevertheless the outlines are true.

However, although I come from the right country, I must also confess my limitations. A psychiatrist does not automatically have the best perspective from which to view primary care. In undertaking primary care research I have had to learn much about the nature of psychiatric disorder and of the requirements for service delivery in that setting. It is important to appreciate this context, for it is different to that of the specialist services, has a different set of problems and a logic of its own.

As a rule, disorder presenting in the primary care setting is mild; it is often non-specific and it is unlabelled. The psychiatrist in his outpatient clinic or private office is in a privileged position in England: at least he is a recipient of a secondary referral, where someone else, usually the GP, has performed a preliminary screening and evaluation, and has tried to channel the patient to the right specialist. Some referrals may be wrongly directed because they are of physical disorder or of mild symptoms which do not require treatment and this may be more so in the United States where the psychiatrist sees many more cases by self-referral, but, by and large, he starts with a given framework in which to commence his assessment and knows where to concentrate his efforts.

In contrast, the general practitioner starts not knowing, as any new patient arrives, whether he has cancer, eyestrain, a pain due to depression, a minor worry about his health best managed by reassurance, or a covert presentation of someone else's problem, such as an apparently sick child which masks the mother's own worries about something else. One must have great respect for the GP's skills in mastering this task.

There is another well-known difference to the psychiatrist. He has on average about 50 minutes to assess a new patient, the GP about 7·5 minutes. The first task therefore is to attempt some sorting out in a very short time; what often happens is a provisional assessment, guided by rapidly picking up cues, which is subject to revision if the symptoms persist to a further attendance rather than responding to initial simple measures.

There is also only brief time usually available to the GP for treatment. It is not easy to fit into a crowded surgery session the lengthy procedures of psychiatric treatment. Therefore much of the work which I will present involves the use of various ancillaries rather than the GP to deliver health care in the primary care setting.

An element which, like it or not, will enter into all considerations of primary health care is cost. The primary health care system is cheap in costs to the community, by virtue of its short periods of contact and its absence of inpatient hospital costs. Table 6.1 is derived from a study of community psychiatric nursing which we carried out (Paykel & Griffith, 1983, Mangen et al, 1983). As part of a cost–benefit analysis we costed a variety of items of service for psychiatric patients from the National Health Service and Local Authority Social Services in an area of South London. General practitioner services were the least expensive. In considering innovations in service delivery in primary care their potential addition to this cost may also have to be kept in mind.

Psychiatric disorders share the characteristics of other disorders in general practice: on average they are mild. In a comparison that we carried out of general practice and psychiatric outpatient depressives (Sireling et al., 1985), the general practice patients were less severely ill, and less disturbed on the majority of individual symptom ratings. On Research Diagnostic Criteria (Spitzer et al., 1978) they were less likely to be major depressives, and if major were less likely to fit criteria for primary, endogenous, retarded, simple and situational subtypes; most

Table 6.1 *Representative costs of some services in the National Health Service.*

	Unit	Cost (£'s)
Nonpsychiatric hospital treatment		
Inpatient	Week	245·70
Day patient	Week	33·75
Outpatient	1 visit	10·50
Accident and emergency	1 visit	8·15
General practitioner		
Surgery attendance	5 minutes	0·69
Home visit	12 minutes	3·01
Psychiatric facilities		
Inpatient care	Week	92·75
Day patient care	Week	45·75
Psychiatric outpatient attendance		
Consultant psychiatrist	12 minute visit	3·09
Senior registrar	12 minute visit	1·95
Registrar	12 minute visit	1·58
Senior House Officer	12 minute visit	1·36
Clinical psychologist	1 hour visit	6·80
Community psychiatric nurse	1 hour visit	3·95
Psychiatric domiciliary visit		
Consultant psychiatrist	15 minute visit	3·00
Community psychiatric nurse	1·26 hour visit	5·67

From Mangen *et al.* (1983). 1977 prices.

of which reflect more severe and typical depression. Since almost all the studies of what treatments are effective in depression are based on outpatients or inpatients treated by psychiatrists, there are clearly large gaps in our knowledge of whether standard treatments convey any great advantage over natural remission in primary care settings.

The natural history of the milder psychiatric disorders in primary care also remains to be studied adequately. The majority of disorders probably have a good outcome and would do so without treatment; a minority of patients show chronic morbidity, some of it severe (Mann *et al.*, 1981) and contribute disproportionately to frequent attendance and the practice load. One group of patients who may not fit in well to primary care conditions are chronic schizophrenics who are poor treatment compliers. Primary care service is demand led and GPs usually assume that if the patient does not re-attend the disorder has remitted, but schizophrenics may require active follow-up and home visits.

Recognition of psychiatric disorder

Goldberg & Huxley (1980) have reviewed the filters and processes involved in treatment and referral of psychiatric disorder in the community. Recognition by the GP is an important factor. Goldberg and his colleagues (Goldberg & Huxley 1980; Marks *et al.* 1979) have studied factors influencing recognition of disorders by GPs in Manchester and Charleston, focussing on the consultation interview. They have divided the variation between doctors into two elements: 'bias' (the tendency of individual doctors towards consistently diagnosing psychiatric disorder) and accuracy (the degree to which the doctor's judgment of the patient as psychiatrically ill corresponds to independent assessment). The two elements were found to be largely independent. Bias related particularly to physicians' empathy, emphasis on psychiatry, sensitivity to verbal cues relating to psychological disorders, and to being a lower status doctor. Accuracy of diagnosis was determined more by interview skills and academic ability.

The factors studied by this group involve qualities of the doctor. Factors in the patient and the disorder have received less study. We studied factors in the patient with one disorder, depression, specifically by comparing patients with RDC major depression recognized by the GP with those unrecognized in the consultation but identified by subsequent screening by the GHQ and interview by a psychiatrist (Freeling *et al.*, 1985). About half the major depressives presenting were unrecognized. Comparing data obtained at psychiatric interview on both groups, what was most remarkable was a relative absence of differences, but there were some meaningful differences. Unrecognized depressives had less overt depressive symptoms: less overt depressed mood and depressed appearance, less insight; they had been depressed for longer, and were more likely to have a depression related to physical illness.

The British history of attempts to improve GP psychological awareness goes back to the group case seminar approach of Michael Balint (Balint, 1957) focussing on the doctor–patient interaction. Subsequent early work at the Tavistock clinic involved attachment of social workers and others in primary care.

The modern innovation has been the introduction of explicit programmes of vocational training which have become obligatory for trainee general practitioners. Such programmes lay considerable emphasis on identification of psychological problems and use of counselling techniques. Each year, at present, about 1,000 vocationally trained general practitioners join the pool of 22,000 general practitioners. By the year 2000, 70% of British GPs will have been through such schemes (P. Freeling, personal communication) and will also have been medical students at a time when there has been much more psychiatry in medical school teaching than in an earlier era. The scene is changing and all the studies of recognition may become outmoded.

Goldberg *et al.* (1980) have described an educational experiment. Family practice residents in Charleston, South Carolina, who were ranked poorly in recognition of psychiatric disorder were randomly assigned to receive four 45-minute special instructional sessions based on videotapes of their own consultations. The index group showed significant improvement in recognition. In a study in the United Kingdom, peer review of videotaped interviews by experienced GPs improved general interview techniques in relation to a comparison group (Verby *et al.*, 1979).

Better recognition of disorders would not necessarily bring benefit. Screening and recognition of mild disorders may not have much point to it if the spontaneous prognosis is in any case good, or GP's therapeutic interventions are of little benefit. Johnstone & Goldberg (1976) reported a study in which the patients of Johnstone, a general practitioner, received the General Health Questionnaire and he was informed of GHQ scores for half. Patients found on reassessment to have psychiatric disorder were compared at follow-up after one year with high GHQ scorers of whom the GP was not informed, and with patients diagnosed by the GP at initial assessment as having psychiatric disorder. The index cases showed a course closely comparable to controls with recognized morbidity, and significantly better than those with unrecognized morbidity, in duration of disturbance during the study year, proportion judged well at follow up and GHQ scores at follow up. The better outcome on GHQ scores only applied to severe disorders: mild disorders did well even if unrecognized. These findings suggest that recognition of disorder, leading to subsequent treatment, is beneficial. However, Hoeper *et al.* (1984) in the USA did not find that feeding back GHQ results to primary care physicians increased detection rates for mental illness.

Psychotropic drugs in primary care

Before evaluating alternative treatment techniques in primary care, it is necessary to consider drug treatment. GPs have been criticized on the one hand, as uncritical purveyors of pills for personal problems (Trethowan, 1975) and on the other as inaccurate prescribers who underuse antidepressants (Tyrer, 1978).

A distinction must be made between antidepressants and benzodiazepine minor tranquilizers. Tricyclic antidepressants do not produce any major problems of dependence. The major question has concerned efficacy: are they effective in the mild and often transient depressions treated in primary care? Studies have shown them superior to placebo in general practice in Australia (Blashki *et al.*, 1971) Scotland (Thomson *et al.*, 1982) and the USA (Rickels *et al.*, 1973). However, the available studies have often been in the more severe spectrum of general practice depressives, or in samples not well characterized and without attempts to distinguish characteristics of those who show the drug placebo differences.

We have therefore undertaken a double blind controlled trial of amitriptyline versus placebo in a heterogenous sample of general practice depressives Paykel *et al.* (1988), with particular emphasis on obtaining a relatively mild sample. One hundred and forty one general practice depressives were treated for six weeks (minimum of four weeks) with amitriptyline (median dose 125 mg daily) versus placebo. We found surprisingly strong drug effects, starting to appear as early as two weeks, strong and consistent by six weeks. Symptoms affected were core symptoms of depression. Extensive analyses were undertaken to seek responsive and unresponsive subgroups. Classifications were related to severity, endogenous symptoms, presence of stress, demographic and history variables which have been suggested to influence outcome. Drug was superior to placebo in virtually all groups, the exception being depressives only fitting criteria for RDC minor rather than major depression, and those of lower initial severity, below 13 on the 17-item Hamilton Scale for Depression.

These findings suggest that the overall benefit of antidepressant drugs is substantial. They are economical treatments, not time-consuming for the doctor, and may be a yardstick against which other treatments must be measured. There is evidence that cognitive therapy is as effective as drug treatments for depression in primary care (Blackburn et al., 1981; Teasdale et al., 1984) but it is much more expensive in therapist time. However, since often GPs' information on correct use of the drugs is limited, our findings do suggest the potential value of programs of GP education aimed at appropriate prescribing.

The issues with benzodiazepines are different. The potential for low-grade dependence is now well recognised (Petursson & Lader, 1981). Figures for consumption in the general population, especially by females, are quite high: in the United States in 1979 14·1% of women and 7·5% of men had had antianxiety agents in the last year (Mellinger & Balter, 1981) and figures for the United Kingdom are comparable (Balter et al. 1974). Effectiveness for minor anxiety or depression is at best palliative and probably short term.

Catalan et al. (1984) described a controlled trial in which patients with a new episode of minor affective disorder, predominantly anxiety, to whom GPs would normally have prescribed anxiolytic medications were randomly assigned to receive either these or brief counselling from the GPs at the initial session. Withholding of medication proved feasible and only involved a mean of two minutes extra at the initial consultation (mean 12 vs. 10·5 minutes, difference NS). There were no subsequent differences in the number of consultations, levels of symptoms or social adjustment. Withholding drugs did not prolong psychological distress, increase consumption of alcohol, tobacco and other drugs, lead to patient dissatisfaction, or make unreasonable demands on the general practitioners' time.

Counselling and psychotherapeutic techniques

GPs' verbal treatments for psychiatric disorder tend to involve didactic advice rather than psychotherapeutic or interpretive techniques (Brodaty et al., 1982). Can GPs usefully employ counselling and interpretive psychotherapy? There are two potential restraints: training and the time available to apply such techniques in the conditions of general practice. The time problem can be solved by the setting aside of some longer surgery appointments outside the busiest consultation hours.

Counselling techniques, with an emphasis on brief pragmatic rather than deeply interpretive methods, can be taught to GPs. Long *et al.* (1976) have described a training course with this aim. Bendix (1982) has published a detailed manual for GPs, describing a psychotherapeutic technique depending on reflection of statements and clarification.

An alternative is the attachment of trained counsellors to work in primary care. There is a growing literature on such attachments, and a growing interest by British GPs in having such workers attached (Waydenfeld & Waydenfeld 1980).

Effectiveness of such interventions has not yet been demonstrated. Ashurst (1983) has described an experiment in which patients in practices in the city of Southampton and in a county town were randomly assigned to see counsellors. Effects of counselling were disappointing. There was little difference between the two groups on symptoms, prescribing of drugs, or consultation time with GPs. Brodaty & Andrews (1983) randomly assigned patients in primary care to brief psychotherapy from a psychiatrist, discussion of problems with the GP for eight weekly sessions of half an hour each, and no treatment. There were no differences in symptoms or social outcome, but the samples (18 per treatment group) were small.

Psychiatric nurses

Perhaps the most innovative and best-evaluated approaches in primary care have involved psychiatric nurses. The most direct applications to primary care have come from the work of Isaac Marks and colleagues. In the 1970s they pioneered the training of psychiatric nurses to apply behavioural methods of treatment, particularly to patients with phobias, obsessive-compulsive and sexual disorders (Marks *et al.*, 1973). Such nurses were as effective as psychologists and psychiatrists in treating phobias (Marks *et al.*, 1975) and a costing exercise suggested cost-effectiveness (Ginsberg & Marks, 1977).

Later they explored the value of such nurse therapists in primary care, in a randomised controlled trial (Marks 1985 *a, b*). Ninety-two patients from four general practices, mainly with phobic or obsessive–compulsive disorders, were randomly allocated to treatment from nurse therapists, or to a control year on a waiting list during which they received usual care from GPs. Disorders were relatively chronic, with a mean problem duration of seven years. Treated patients, who received a mean of seven treatment sessions, showed highly significant improvement compared with controls at six and 12 months. Control patients received behaviour therapy after a year, and then improved dramatically. In a cost–benefit analysis, treated patients decreased their use of resources by a mean of £14 compared with the previous year, while untreated patients increased by £131, mainly due to more absences from work, more hospital treatment and drugs (Ginsberg *et al.*, 1984). The authors estimated that, if benefits lasted for two years, and if a nurse could treat 46 patients year, then it would be cheaper for the community to give such patients nurse behavioural therapy rather than withhold it.

This was a very well-evaluated innovative program with clear aims. Only about 1 % of surgery attenders were regarded by GPs as having problems suitable for behaviour therapy but, as in other similar studies, a substantial proportion of suitable cases were also found to be missed by GPs. The authors estimated that one full-time nurse could usefully serve a primary care population of 30,000.

In the late 1970s we studied treatment by another group of psychiatric nurses: community psychiatric nurses. These have been a burgeoning specialty in Britain since the early 1970s, and have come to be an essential component of a psychiatric service. Qualified psychiatric nurses, with some additional training in community approaches, usually work in association with psychiatric specialist teams, particularly in the follow-up care of schizophrenics. Some work instead in primary care (Corser & Ryce, 1977).

Our evaluative study involved nurses in psychiatric teams rather than in primary care, but with a somewhat similar patient group, relatively chronic neurotic patients with mild symptoms but considerable social impairment. Patients were randomly assigned to community psychiatric nurses as key-workers, or to continue to see psychiatrists as outpatients. Ninety one patients completed at least six months in the study design and 71 patients 18 months (Paykel *et al.*, 1982; Paykel & Griffith, 1983; Mangen *et al.*, 1983). Nursing care was of equal efficacy to care from psychiatrists in terms of symptoms, social function and family burden. Consumer satisfaction was higher in the group treated by nurses. Nursing care was mainly at home and often involved contact with relatives; the predominant modality was supportive psychotherapy. Nurses initially saw their patients more frequently than psychiatrists but adopted a well-structured approach with goal setting, and achieved more discharges in a service which was cheaper than care from psychiatrists. The model of care was less specific than Marks' behavioural psychotherapy but would appear to be suitable for a variety of neurotic patients.

The picture is not all one-sided. Psychiatrists have criticized the diversion of psychiatric nurses to work with milder patients rather than the more severely ill chronically disabled schizophrenics whom staff often find less attractive and, in a resource-starved service, have feared the loss of a valuable service. Wooff *et al* (1986) studied the community psychiatric nursing service in Salford, predominantly located in primary care. The establishment of the service corresponded to an increase in prevalence of treated disorder, apparently due to an increase in the case-load of patients with primary care morbidity, without any consequent sparing of the specialist services. In a more intensive study (K. Wooff, personal communication) the author found a number of problems, including poor links with the specialist psychiatric services and with primary care workers other than the GP, a lack of systematic supervision, and some evidence of poor interpersonal interviewing skills.

Critics of psychiatric nursing in primary care may miss the point that there is a clientele with legitimate needs which may not at present be well served, but the problem of allocation of scarce resources is a real and familiar one. In the United Kingdom, specialist services and primary care are funded separately and a solution might be to arrange the funding of primary care psychiatric nurses from the primary care resources rather than from the specialist services, from which they are funded at the moment. The studies do not necessarily indicate that nurses are better than other professionals, and similar arrangements might need to be applied to other groups. What is clear is that skilled and focussed professional time applied in general practice can produce good results.

Social workers

Social workers have a specific set of skills, overlapping with those of other psychiatric workers, but distinct from them. Attachment of social workers to primary care might be a useful way of serving the substantial proportion of general practice attenders for whom psychiatric symptoms are interwoven with social and personal problems.

Cooper *et al.* (1975) described a study in which a social worker was attached to a metropolitan London practice. The workers regarded random assignment as impractical and drew a control sample from similar practices lacking social work. They found trends for less use of medication and less referral to psychiatric and social agencies in the group receiving social work, and significantly greater improvement in symptoms and social adjustment. Most of the patients had neurotic disorders. Two-thirds of the social work time was devoted to practical helping activities and only one-quarter to more clear-cut casework (Shepherd *et al.*, 1979). There was a tendency for unmarried patients to be referred to the social worker but beneficial effects tended to be most prominent on the marital relationship, in married patients.

It is difficult to be confident in comparisons with control groups not randomly assigned, since it is not easy to match for all possible covert selection factors. Seven or eight years later the same research unit found random assignment feasible. Corney (1984) studied depressed women aged 18–45, who had been found to constitute a high proportion of referrals to attached social workers. Women were randomly assigned to social workers and to routine treatment by GPs and were reassessed six months later. There were few differences in clinical and social outcome or use of psychotropic drugs, but in women with acute or chronic depression associated with major marital problems there was evidence of benefit on symptoms and social adjustment. Again, a major component of the work was found to be practical social help.

Clinical Psychologists

Clinical psychologists are another professional group with a potential role in primary care. Clinical psychology in Britain has concentrated on behavioural approaches, although psychotherapeutic and, to an increasing extent, cognitive approaches are also employed.

For about ten years, occasional reports of work by clinical psychologists in primary care have been appearing (France & Robson 1982). Earll & Kincey (1982) reported the first controlled comparison with routine general practice management, using relatively small samples. They found a short-term reduction in use of psychotropic drugs during the treatment period but no reduction in GP consultation and no longer-term significant difference.

Robson et al. (1984) randomly assigned 429 patients, predominantly with anxiety, interpersonal problems, depression and habit disorders to a behaviourally oriented primary care clinical psychology service for up to 10 weeks, (mean of 3·7 sessions, 2·5 hours), or to routine general practice care. There were significant advantages in the clinical psychology group on problem severity, effect on sufferer and household, number of visits to GP between ten weeks and six months, and costs of psychotropic drugs prescribed. The nature of the psychological intervention was not clearly described, nor was its cost evaluated.

Psychiatrists in primary care

If the psychiatric nurse, social worker and psychologist, why not the psychiatrist? A relatively new phenomenon in Britain has been of psychiatrists themselves going out from the hospital or consulting room, to work in primary care settings, most commonly health centres or group practices. Strathdee & Williams (1984) caught the mood of this development nicely with the title of an article 'The silent growth of a new service'. In a survey of psychiatrists they carried out in 1982 about one-fifth indicated that they, or their junior staff, did some work in a general practice setting. Since then there has been further growth. The work generates considerable enthusiasm, with particular advantages being seen by the psychiatrists involved in it including improved liaison with the primary health care team, easier access to background information, ability to involve the GP in treatment, earlier referral, prevention of hospital admission and continuity of care. Such work appears to take place most commonly in two rural regions, the West country and East Anglia, less so in London. My own experience suggests that it is particularly suitable to rural areas where psychiatric outpatient clinics are long distances from many of the patients, with formidable public transport difficulties.

There are different patterns of work. In the survey by Strathdee & Williams, 64% of psychiatrists in the general practice setting assessed and treated patients using either what the authors termed the 'shifted outpatient clinic' pattern, where the format of work was similar to the hospital outpatient clinic, or the 'liaison attachment' pattern, where the psychiatrist had instituted working links and training with other professionals such as social workers, psychologists and community psychiatric nurses.

Of the psychiatrists, 28% used a different mode of working – the 'consultation' pattern. For psychotherapeutically oriented psychiatrists this comprised Balint-style seminars discussing the doctor–patient relationship; for the less psychotherapeutic, the assessment of patients, often in collaboration with the GP, who then took on the treatment. The essential element here is the working by advice and discussion with GPs rather than predominantly by direct care.

This new movement has now yet been evaluated critically in terms of cost-effectiveness. There is no doubt of its continuing growth, or of the enthusiasm it generates in younger psychiatrists.

Prevention

In theory, primary care physicians are well placed to undertake a role in prevention, at least in so far as early case detection and early intervention are concerned. A few years ago a working party of general practitioners, including two psychiatrists, examined some of the possibilities (Royal College of General Practitioners, 1981). These ranged from child rearing and child care, to attempted suicide and problem drinking.

In spite of good intentions, a note of caution must be sounded. The difficulties in effective prevention of psychiatric disorder are formidable in the present state of knowledge. Most psychiatric disorders appear to be heavily multifactorial in aetiology: prevention aimed at single factors, even if effective, will have a small and not easily shown effect on many disorders rather than a single clear effect on one. Ideas for intervention tend to evolve into general prescriptions for good living, good motherhood and the like which are highly desirable but not easily achievable in the face of practical human realities. The proportional of mild disorders which evolve into severe ones is not known but it is probably small; if that is the case and most mild disorders have a good outcome, early intervention will not be cost-effective. At present, it is hard to point to any programme which has clearly been shown to be effective in preventing mental illness, other than mental retardation. Failing this, a heavy investment of resources on prevention in primary care would be unwise, but small, carefully evaluated projects would be timely.

Conclusions

This paper has looked at service developments and innovations in care of mental disorders in primary care in a number of different areas, ranging over a spectrum of recognition of disorder, treatment by drugs, counselling by GPs and others, and use of a variety of other personnel in the primary care setting.

Two background issues are important. The first is the nature of the relatively mild nonspecific, early and masked disorder which predominates in primary care. The second is the nature of the primary care presentation, where the first task is to sort the important from the nonimportant and this may be gradual and staged, with gradual deployment of more major intervention as the disorder crystallises, usually accompanied all the way through by time constraints.

I have confined myself largely to British reports, partly because of the theme of this volume and partly because of the well developed state of British primary care. This limitation reflects something wider: most of the literature on primary care psychiatry is from well developed Western countries with well resourced health care systems. Primary care psychiatry is much more important for less developed countries: it is the only psychiatry for the majority of the population, unless they are extremely ill. Yet much less has been written about this situation, and for this paper it has seemed best not to touch on it.

Some of the innovations described in this paper involved sharpening the skills of the GP himself, but more involve deployment of other professionals into the primary care team. I think that this is the most likely way forward, at least in the British system. It needs to be done with a clear head: it really involves an interpenetration of generalised primary care and specialist secondary referral roles into the same setting, and both sides need to evaluate coolly the benefits and costs. The GP may lose one of the benefits usually associated with primary care: the ability to comprehend knowledge of the whole person and continuity of care within a single carer. The specialist worker is in danger of getting out of his depth and uncritically applying the techniques for disorders which are severe to those which are mild.

These interventions therefore require careful evaluation. Overall, the best evaluations and the clearest demonstrations of benefit have been with the various disciplines applying behavioural therapies. They have always been among the best evaluators and their targeted approach lends itself well to the evaluation of effectiveness. However, the behavioural techniques are at present applicable only to a minority of psychiatric disorders in general practice, and even here evaluations of cost effectiveness against drug therapies or against deploying the same personnel for the severely disordered have not much been attempted. There is unquestionably a large field of further evaluative studies in primary care psychiatric treatment still to be carried out. The issues are not only efficacy but cost and some value-laden questions of the best deployment of limited resources. The focus of studies in primary care psychiatry is at present turning very much towards treatment approaches, and this is likely to continue.

References

Ashurst, P. M. (1983). Evaluation of counselling in a general practice setting: preliminary communication. *Journal of the Royal College of Medicine*, **72**, 657–9.

Balint, M. (1957). *The Doctor, His Patient and the Illness*. London, Pitman.

Balter, M. B., Levine, J. & Manheimer, D. I. (1974). Cross-National study of the extent of anti anxiety/sedative drug use. *New England Journal of Medicine*. **390**, 769–74.

Bendix, T. (1982). The anxious patient: the therapeutic dialogue in clinical practice. In H. J. Wright, (ed.) translated M. Schou, D. N. Skow & D. Henderson) Edinburgh: Churchill Livingstone.

Blackburn, I. M., Bishop, S., Glen, A. I. M., Whalley, L. J. & Christie, J. E. (1981). The efficacy of cognitive therapy in depression: a treatment trial using cognitive therapy and pharmacotherpay, each alone and in combination. *British Journal of Psychiatry*, **139**, 181–9.

Blashki, T. G., Mowbray, R. & Davies, B. (1971). Controlled trial of amitriptyline in general practice. *British Medical Journal*, **1**, 133–8.

Brodaty, H., Andrews, G. & Austin, A. (1982). Psychiatric illness in general practice II: How is it managed? *Australian Family Physician*, **11**, 682–6.

Brodaty, H. & Andrews, G. Brief psychotherapy in family practice. (1983), A controlled prospective intervention trial. *British Journal of Psychiatry*, **143**, 11–19.

Catalan, J., Gath, D., Edmonds, G., & Ennis, J. (1984). The effects of non-prescribing of anxiolytics in general practice. Controlled evaluation of psychiatric and social outcome. *British Journal of Psychiatry*, **144**, 593–602.

Cooper, B., Harwin, B. G., Depla, C. & Shepherd, M. (1975). Mental health care in the community: an evaluative study. *Psychological Medicine* **5**, 372–80.

Corney, R. H. (1984). The effectiveness of attached social workers in the management of depressed female patients in general practice. *Psychological Medicine Monograph Supplement* **6**.

Corser, C. M. & Ryce, S. W. (1977). Community mental health care: a model based on the primary care team. *British Medical Journal*, **2**, 936–8.

Earll, L. & Kincey, J. (1982). Clinical psychology in general practice: a controlled trial evaluation. *Journal of the Royal College of General Practice*, **32**, 32–7.

France, R. & Robson, M. (1982). Work of the clinical psychologist in general practice: preliminary communication. *Journal of the Royal Society of Medicine* **75**, 185–9.

Freeling, P., Rao, B. M., Paykel, E. S., Sireling, L. I. & Burton, R. H. (1985). Unrecognised depression in general practice. *British Medical Journal*, **290**, 1880–3.

Ginsberg, G. & Marks, I. (1977). Costs and benefits of behavioural psychotherapy:

a pilot study of neurotics treated by nurse-therapists. *Psychological Medicine* **7**, 685–700.

Ginsberg, G., Marks, I. & Waters, H. (1984). Cost–benefit analysis of a controlled trial of nurse therapy for neuroses in primary care. *Psychological Medicine*, **14**, 683–90.

Goldberg, D. P., & Huxley, P. Mental illness in the community. London: Tavistock (1980).

Goldberg, D. P., Steele, J. J., Smith, C. & Spivey, L. (1980). Training family doctors to recognise psychiatric illness with increased accuracy. *Lancet*, 521–3.

Hoeper, E. W., Kessler, L. G., Nycz, G. R., Burke, J. D. Jr & Pierce, W. E. (1984). The usefulness of screening for mental illness. *Lancet*, 33–5 (1984)

Johnstone, A. & Goldberg, D. P. (1976). Psychiatric screening in general practice: a controlled trial. *Lancet*, 605–8.

Long, B. E. L., Harris, C. M. & Byrne, P. S. (1976). A method of teaching counselling. *Medical Education*, **10**, 198–204.

Mangen, S. P., Paykel, E. S., Griffith, J. H., Burchell, A. & Mancini, P. (1983). Cost effectiveness of community psychiatric nurse or outpatient psychiatrist care of neurotic patients. *Psychological Medicine* **13**, 401–16.

Mann, A. H., Jenkins, R. & Belsey, E. (1981). The twelve-month outcome of patients with neurotic illness in general practice. *Psychological Medicine*, **11**, 535–50.

Marks, I. M. (1985 a). Psychiatric nurse therapists in primary care. Book in *Research Series of Royal College of Nursing*, London.

Marks, I. M. (1985 b). Controlled trial of psychiatric nurse therapists in primary care. *British Medical Journal*, **290**, 1181–4.

Marks, I. M., Connolly, J. & Hallam, R. S. (1973). Psychiatric nurse as therapist. *British Medical Journal*, **3**, 156–60.

Marks, I. M., Hallam, R. S., PhilPott, R. & Connolly, J. C. (1975). Nurse therapists in behavioural psychotherapy. *British Medical Journal*, **3**, 144–8.

Marks, J. N., Goldberg, D. P. & Hillier, V. F. (1979). Determinants of the ability of general practitioners to detect psychiatric illness. *Psychological Medicine* **9**, 337–53.

Mellinger, G. D. & Balter, M. B. (1981). Prevalence and pattern of use of psychotherapeutic drugs: results from a 1979 National Survey of American Adults. In: *Impact of Psychotropic Drugs*. (Tognoni, G., Ballantuona, C. & Lader, M. eds) Elsevier, North Holland Biomedical Press.

Paykel, E. S., Mangen, S. P., Griffiths, J. H. & Burns, T. P. (1982). Community psychiatric nursing for neurotic patients: a controlled trial. *British Journal of Psychiatry*, **140**, 573–81.

Paykel, E. S. & Griffiths, J. H. (1983). Community psychiatric nursing for neurotic patients: the Springfield controlled trial. *Research Monographs in Nursing Series*. Royal College of Nursing, London

Paykel, E. S., Hollyman, J. A., Freeling, P. & Sedgwick, P. (1988). Predictors of therapeutic benefit from amitriptyline in mild depression: a general practice placebo-controlled trial. *J. Affective Disorder*, **14**, 83–95.

Petursson, H. & Lader, M. H. (1981). Withdrawal from long-term benzodiazepine treatment. *British Medical Journal*, **283**, 643–5.

Rickels, K., Gordon, P. E., Wheeler Jenkins, B., Parloff, M., Sachs, T. & Stepansky, W. (1973). Drug treatment in depressive illness (amitriptyline and chlordiazepoxide in two neurotic populations). *Diseases of the Nervous System*, **31**, 30–42.

Robson, M., France, R. & Bland, M. (1984). Clinical psychologist in primary care: controlled clinical and economic evaluation. *British Medical Journal*, **288**, 1805–8.

Royal College of General Practitioners. (1981). Prevention of psychiatric disorders in general practice. *Report from general practice* **20**. RCGP, London.

Shepherd, M, Harwin, B. G., Depla, C. & Cairns, V. (1979). Social work and the primary care of mental disorder. *Psychological Medicine*, **9**, 661–9.

Sireling, L. I., Freeling, P., Paykel, E. S. & Rao, B. M. (1985). Depression in general practice: clinical features and comparison with out-patients. *British Journal of Psychiatry*, **147**, 119–27.

Spitzer, R. L., Endicott, J. & Robins, E. (1978). Research Diagnostic Criteria: rationale and reliability. *Archives of General Psychiatry* **35**, 773–82.

Strathdee, G. & Williams, P. (1984). A survey of psychiatrists in primary care: the silent growth of a new service. *Journal of the Royal College of General Practice* **34**, 615–18.

Teasdale, J. D., Fennell, M. J. V., Hibbert, G. A. & Amies, P. L. (1984). Cognitive therapy for major depressive disorder in primary care. *British Journal of Psychiatry*, **144**, 400–6.

Thomson, J., Rankin, H., Ashcroft, G. W., Yats, C. M., McQueen, J. K. & Cummings, S. W. (1982). The treatment of depression in general practice: a comparison of L-tryptophan, amitriptyline and a combination of L-tryptophan and amitriptyline with placebo. *Psychological Medicine*, **12**, 741–51.

Trethowan, W. H. (1975). Pills for personal problems. *British Medical Journal* **3**, 749–51.

Tyrer, P. (1978). Drug treatment of psychiatric patients in general practice. *British Medical Journal*, **2**, 1008–10.

Verby, J. E., Holden, P. & Davis, R. H. (1979). Peer review of consultations in primary care: the use of audiovisual recordings. *British Medical Journal* **1**, 1686–8.

Waydenfeld, D. & Waydenfeld, S. W. (1980). Counselling in general practice. *Journal of the Royal College of General Practice*, **30**, 671–7.

Wooff, K., Goldberg, D. P. & Fryers, T. (1986). Patients in receipt of community psychiatric nursing care in Salford 1976–1982. *Psychological Medicine* **16**, 407–14.

Section C: Emergency services

Editors' Commentary

Innovative emergency and crisis intervention services have spread in many countries. Their potential may include a decrease in admission rates and perhaps in suicide attempts. In this section Katschnig & Konieczna survey the wide variety of emergency services that have sprung up in Europe. All offer 'no waiting-list psychiatry'. The clients served include those in psychosocial crisis, acute psychotic patients, and recently chronic psychotic patients living in the community. Staff must be able to diagnose a wide range of problems and to be skilful in dealing with violence.

Emergency services come in many forms ranging from a hot-line telephone which protects the caller's anonymity, to staff readily available in a clinic or hospital, to a mobile team which visits subjects at home or wherever else the crisis presents. There are different tradeoffs to the various sites of care, different population sizes served, and different professional mixes of staff manning the emergency service.

In recent years there has been a tendency to include emergency care as one of many responsibilities for community mental health centres which are increasingly being set up in Europe. Katschnig & Konieczna contrast the pros and cons of this comprehensive approach with those of providing specialized services. Some places have both types of service, creating substantial tension.

Segal notes that in the USA emergency services reside largely in psychiatric emergency rooms in the general hospital. He distinguishes substitutive services for crisis, which withdraw the patient from the crisis pressure, from supplemental (supportive) services which maintain sufferers in their life situation, and cites 'neighbourhood watch' schemes as an example of the latter.

7

Innovative approaches to delivery of emergency services in Europe

Heinz Katschnig & Terese Konieczna

This paper is based on our knowledge of a wide variety of psychiatric emergency and crisis intervention services in the European region of the World Health Organization. It is, however, safe to assume that a number of conclusions reached are also valid for the United States, since – with the exception of the United Kingdom and some other countries, especially in Eastern Europe – the health care structure of many European countries resembles that of the United States.

Fifteen years ago in many places in Europe the traditional pattern of psychiatric care, relying on a distant large mental hospital caring mainly for psychotic patients and on psychiatrists in private practice focussing on neurotic and emotional disorders, was still dominant. With some exceptions – among them the United Kingdom – innovative approaches to psychiatric care were largely unknown. Today, however, we see a motley picture of traditional and new psychiatric services, including those for emergency care and crisis intervention. In Europe, the pattern of psychiatric services has always varied across countries due to different financial, legal, organizational and professional conditions, the introduction of community psychiatric services at different times in different countries, and even in different parts of the same country. In Austria we can find an advanced community psychiatric care system in a small province with 400,000 inhabitants alongside a traditional mental hospital-based psychiatric service in a neighbouring province of equal population size.

One general observation can, however, be made: wherever community psychiatry has been introduced in Europe, it has been mainly concerned with rehabilitation, i.e. the transition from psychiatric care back to society. Emergency psychiatry and crisis intervention concern the reverse transition, from society into psychiatric care, and have been relatively neglected in planning, being simply regarded as one of many aspects of traditional psychiatric care.

Despite this backlog of planned emergency psychiatric services, an increasing number of local initiatives have been seen in the last 15 years to meet the apparent but hitherto neglected need for such services. No uniform pattern of such services exists across different European countries or within one country, and within towns and districts different types of services have been developed and co-exist. Different theoretical backgrounds and goals of those setting up a service locally are partly responsible for this confusing picture.

These goals are similar to those in the United States. They include suicide prevention and crisis intervention, the prevention of hospitalization, or at least replacement of the traditional 'hard landing' in psychiatric institutions by a 'smooth landing'. In several instances the creation of a psychiatric emergency service was a pragmatic reaction to the increasing demand for emergency care by chronic psychotic patients who, due to the de-institutionalization programs today live to a large extent in the community. These historical roots of crisis intervention and psychiatric emergency services are described elsewhere in more detail (Katschnig *et al.*, in press; Katschnig & Cooper, 1988).

Our knowledge of psychiatric emergency and crisis intervention services stems from a survey carried out under the auspices of the Regional Office for Europe of the World Health Organization between 1982 and 1985 in 19 different locations in 12 European countries (Katschnig & Konieczna, in press). This report supplements a previous one by Cooper (1979), who had visited 13 locations in 7 different countries. Altogether 32 locations in 17 European countries were covered, ranging from Great Britain to Bulgaria and from Sweden to Greece, including both Western and Eastern European countries (see Table 7.1).

It has to be stressed that, despite this impressive list, in practically all countries visited, psychiatric emergency services do not yet constitute an integral part of the national psychiatric care system. Furthermore, this field is constantly changing with services disappearing and new ones being created, reflecting the lack of generally agreed guidelines for organizing such services. Altogether, satisfactory emergency psychiatric care is still very rare in Europe.

While the services visited were not really representative of all existing emergency psychiatric services in Europe, they probably include all major types, ranging from psychosocial crisis intervention centres to traditional, purely medical psychiatric emergency wards, from telephone hotlines, to ambulatory and mobile services and to crisis intervention wards, from services specialized in emergency care or crisis intervention to comprehensive systems of psychiatric care where emergency psychiatry is just one component integrated with other components of psychiatric care. From directly observing the daily routine of work, interviews with staff, and publications about their activities, we identified a number of issues which seem

Table 7.1 *Psychiatric emergency and crisis intervention services visited during the WHO Project*

Country	Location
Austria	Vienna
Bulgaria	Sofia
	Pleven
Czechoslovakia	Bratislava
Finland	Helsinki
France	Paris
	Reims
German Democratic Republic	Berlin
Germany, Federal Republic	Münich
	Berlin (West)
	Mannheim
Greece	Athens
Hungary	Budapest
Italy	Trieste
	Perugia
	Arezzo
	Rome
The Netherlands	Amsterdam
	Gröningen
	Utrecht
Poland	Cracow
Spain	Barcelona
Sweden	Linköping
	Stockholm
Switzerland	Zurich
	Berne
	Geneva
Great Britain	London
	Oxford
	Edinburgh
Yugoslavia	Ljubljana
	Belgrade

relevant for planning psychiatric emergency services. We have grouped these issues under three major headings and will illustrate special points using examples of services visited.

The first question concerns the different *subtypes of persons* who need urgent psychiatric help and the implications of such a typology for the adequate provision of services. We will use a typology of persons rather than of problems, although multidimensionality is inherent in any individual's problems. A categorical typology, despite problems of overlap, is better suited to the planning of services.

Second, since we were challenged by the large variety of services encountered we tried to identify some principles by which to clarify them. The site of contact defines the relative position of helper and client, the 'power' structure of their relationship, and the range of possible interactions and interventions; we call this territorial aspect of the contact *'psychosocial topology'*. The pros and cons of telephone hotlines, ambulatory, mobile and overnight stay services will be discussed from this perspective.

Finally, we will discuss a *dilemma* increasingly faced by health planners, the need to choose between specialized and centralized services on the one hand and comprehensive and decentralized services on the other.

Who needs psychiatric emergency care or crisis intervention?

If planning is to be rational, the persons who need psychiatric emergency care or crisis intervention should be defined clearly and their prevalence estimated. However, as in psychiatric diagnosis in general, so in emergency psychiatry terminological and conceptual problems are a major obstacle to progress.

The terms 'psychiatric emergency' and 'crisis' are generally used inter-changeably and with specific meanings. As a specific term, 'psychiatric emergency' usually refers to acute psychotic conditions with suicidal and aggressive behaviour; 'crisis' is usually applied to cases where a psychosocial stress overtaxes the individual's coping ability and leads to distress.

In practice this dichotomy cannot be consistently held up, since pure 'psychosocial crises' are frequently complicated by organic problems (alcohol, drug overdose) and psychotic episodes may well be triggered by life stress events. A multidimensional classification of 'distress syndromes' in need of urgent help – describing psychosocial stressors, psychopathological syndromes, coping resources, organic factors, etc on separate axes – would be more appropriate. For planning purposes simple and categorical classifications are, however, better suited than dimensional ones since they help to focus planning efforts.

Keeping problems of overlap and incomplete coverage in mind we propose a tripartite categorical classification of persons in psychological distress who need urgent professional help.

Patients in acute psychosocial crisis

Such crises usually occur as a consequence of a catastrophic life event. These are often superimposed on an existing personality disorder, chaotic lifestyle, and chronic psychosocial difficulties. The ideal client of crisis intervention centres – someone hit by a severe psychosocial stress but with an otherwise healthy personality and functioning social network – seems rather rare. This means that prolonged psychotherapy is often necessary in addition to acute crisis intervention. Frequently, these people have additional somatic problems due to acute alcohol or drug intake, often with a suicidal intent. In these instances somatic help is needed first.

Patients with acute psychiatric conditions needing urgent medical attention
Here are subsumed acute psychotic episodes of organic or unknown origin and intoxications presenting psychiatric symptoms (alcohol, drugs, overdose or attempted suicide). For such conditions, broad skills are required in assessing psychiatric and somatic conditions and treating them medically. The management of disorganized behaviour, often with suicidal or aggressive components, also requires psychosocial skills.

Chronic psychotic patients living in the community
Due to the deinstitutionalization movement such patients are increasingly asking for emergency help in general medical and psychiatric services. This population is at high risk of overreacting to ordinary psychosocial stressors. In most of these patients medical (partly due to long-term medication), psychological and social problems may present simultaneously – with an emphasis on the latter two – so a mixture of all the appropriate skills is necessary to provide adequate help in times of instability and crisis.

No precise epidemiological figures are available on the incidence of psychiatric emergencies and crises in the general population let alone on the three subpopulations just delineated. For the United States Klerman (1985) estimates that due to adverse life events, in one year approximately 50 million persons experience distressing emotional symptoms – but not necessarily a definable and diagnosable mental illness; 30–35 million people are estimated as having a definable psychiatric disorder, but there are no indications of the prevalence of emergencies in this population. Among the 30–35 million mentally ill in the United States about 1–2 million have chronic mental illness and extensive social disability, an unknown proportion of whom are prone to become unstable and need urgent intervention. Kaskey & Ianzito (1984) suggest that emergencies among chronic psychotic patients in the community are increasing in frequency: for a Massachusetts catchment area of about 500,000 inhabitants the number of psychiatric emergencies in the general hospital emergency room rose from less than 100 to about 2,600 per year from 1972 to 1982; during the same period, the state hospital population of this catchment area declined from 2,500 to 250 patients.

The relative proportions of the three different types of patients among attenders of a specific service depend on the patients' self-concept, designation of the service, its mode of financing, and other influences on the selection of clients. We will come back to these factors below when discussing different types of services.

Expertise in handling these different types of clients and patients is unequally distributed among different professions. Since institutions are often staffed with mainly one type of professional, the provision of adequate help for all three types of clients or patients under one and the same roof may constitute a difficult organizational problem. Since we do not know the distribution of expertise among different professions and services for the various potential clients in distress who want immediate help, all types of services may be confronted with all types of clients, patients and problems, yet only offer a specific type of help based, say, on a crisis theory-oriented self concept or on the medical model. If a person in a psychosocial crisis contacts a psychiatric hospital service, evaluation may be exclusively carried out from the perspective of the medical model, with social network components of such crises tending to be overlooked. Family members may bring a relative who has threatened suicide to a psychiatric hospital and, in so doing, delegate the problem to an outside institution. By threatening suicide, someone may force a doctor to admit him and thus avoid dealing with the problem directly. Hospital doctors are usually not trained well enough to understand such complicated relationships. On the other hand, a schizophrenic living in the community may well present to a crisis intervention centre where his mental illness is overlooked by a young psychologist whose focus of interest is in personal relationships and does not realize that the patient needs neuroleptic medication. Ideally, each service for acute psychological distress should be equipped to deal with the total spectrum of emergency and crisis situations, i.e. with all three types of clients described above.

The proliferation of isolated and specialized services in Europe is obviously not conducive to such a solution. State health systems like the British National Health Service and those in Eastern Europe – due to their financing structure – may find it easier to try out possible solutions to this problem since they can employ a multidisciplinary staff. The Barnet Hospital in North London has for many years had a mobile psychiatrist, a psychiatric nurse and a social worker. This team is available 24 hours a day, 7 days a week and responds to each request for emergency intervention from the community – usually from the general practitioner – within two hours after the call has been received. It provides on-the-spot intervention by all three team members and it appears to work quite efficiently, including for psychogeriatric problems (Ratna, 1982). A further example of such comprehensive psychiatric emergency care can be found in Ljubljana, a town with 190,000 inhabitants in Northern Yugoslavia. There, a community mental health centre works around the clock providing a telephone hotline, outpatient, day-patient and inpatient care and a crisis intervention ward for all types of psychiatric emergencies and crises, with very easy transition from one type of service to another and easy access to all types of professional expertise. Also, easily available under the same roof are full psychiatric inpatient care and aftercare. The provision of such accessible multiprofessional help for persons in distress, who due to their psychological turmoil are unable to judge who best to go to for help, should be a priority in organizing adequate psychiatric emergency services. This issue is related to a more general problem with which psychiatric planners are increasingly confronted in Europe, namely whether emergency psychiatric care and crisis intervention should be offered as a specialized service or as part of the general psychiatric or even medical care system.

In emergency psychiatric services on both sides of the Atlantic, a substantial proportion of clients use these services as a last resort (Bassuk, 1985). These people often have chronic personality disorders and a chaotic lifestyle, lack an available social network or the ability to use an existing one. They are unable to make use of services in a 'normal' way, and wait for an emergency before surmounting the psychological and financial barriers to help (Caroli & Olié, 1979: Häfner-Ranerbauer & Günzler, 1984). These persons tend to turn up repeatedly and so have been called 'chronic crisis patients' (Bassuk & Gerson, 1980) or 'emergency room repeaters' (Walker, 1983), and subgroups have been labelled 'manipulative help rejectors', 'entitled demanders', 'dependent clingers' and 'self-destructive deniers' (Groves, 1978).

While many services complain about 'misuse' by such clients, the question is who should really help them. They cannot cope with their problems in their natural environment and use services which are available around the clock. There may be misuse of emergency services by other health and social services. Not infrequently, emergency psychiatric services complain that other care-givers refer clients too easily, especially outside working hours, when confronted with difficult situations which seem too demanding or if they are unable to organize inpatient admission judged to be necessary. For example, in the emergency service of the Zurich Board of Doctors, three-quarters of all clients to whom the mobile emergency service was called had had unsuccessful contacts with other services. Such 'dumping' (Pisarcik, 1982) is a dilemma for emergency psychiatric services, which cannot easily reject a patient or send him back to the referring institution, and have to cope with his problems themselves.

Dangerousness to self or others needs mention. It is not known what proportion of dangerous patients needing chronic emergency care requires compulsory treatment. The problem of dangerousness due to a psychiatric illness is probably exaggerated by the public; it is a difficult concept and some haruspicy and discrepancy of opinions is always involved in this judgment. The very assumption of dangerousness and the initiation of psychiatric intervention may lead to a self-fulfilling prophecy contributing to violent behaviour. Techniques to defuse such escalation are most important and should be taught more widely (Everstine & Everstine, 1983).

While it is difficult to prove the validity of a prediction of dangerousness, according to the laws of most countries such an assumption leads to compulsory admission. Though clinicians make quite consistent decisions about dangerousness to self or others, in quite a few cases 'even experienced and highly trained clinicians don't respond in an equitable manner' (Segal *et al.*, 1985).

Types of services – the 'psychosocial topology' of psychiatric emergency contacts

In Europe psychiatric care is usually regarded as something to be avoided. Although psychoanalysis and psychotherapy originated in Europe, the public perceives today's psychiatry as dealing largely with mental illness proper rather than with life problems. Contact with a psychiatrist means substantial stigma and is therefore avoided as long as possible. Unfortunately, many general practitioners and other doctors share the same prejudices of lay people and resist referring patients to psychiatrists.

This stigma has two implications for the adequate provision of professional crisis or emergency services: first, psychological and psychiatric problems may become very severe, possibly to the point where compulsory measures are unavoidable, before specialized psychiatric help is sought. Secondly, in patients who preserve some judgment despite great psychological distress, the possible stigma from contacting a psychiatric service may be important. It is unclear whether the more pronounced inclination of American psychiatry to psychotherapy reduces the stigma for potential clients of emergency services in the United States. European planners of psychiatric emergency or crisis intervention services had to consider this reluctance of the public to get in touch with psychiatry. The large variety of types of services encountered in the 17 European countries during the WHO project reflect different responses to this reluctance.

As mentioned, 'psychosocial topology' refers to the complex geographical, organizational and psychological relationships between clients and helpers. The *place* where contact is made between the persons needing help and those providing it, is central to the acceptability of help by the client to the kind of help that can be provided. How easy it is for the potential client to withdraw before the help reaches a degree he does not want, e.g. compulsory admission to a mental hospital – intimately depends on physical and other aspects of the contact, e.g. whether contact is made by telephone or by face-to-face contact; whether the encounter is on the premises of a service or in a person's home; who calls in a mobile emergency team; and finally, whether the person is transported against his/her will to a psychiatric institution.

Four different 'topological' service settings can be distinguished in the contact between client and service: telephone, outpatients (client comes to service), mobile (service goes to client), and overnight stay (client comes or is brought to service and remains). In any single case, several of these services may be used in turn. Telephone contacts have special importance as a universal means of access to all other types of services.

Other ways of classifying helping facilities for psychiatric emergencies and crises are also possible. Segal distinguishes substitutive, supportive and supplemental facilities (this volume, page 106). We could also separate medically oriented emergency services from more psychosocially inspired crisis intervention services. Instead, we have chosen the site of contact to classify the services, since it focuses on a paramount characteristic of emergency contacts, the transition from the community to psychiatric care.

Telephone services

The main advantage of the telephone in emergency psychiatry is its accessibility. The threshold for using the phone is comparatively low because the caller can remain anonymous and does not need to be afraid of being labelled as a psychiatric case or even hospitalized. The caller remains in control on his own 'territory' at a secure distance from the professionals. However, for the helper, contacts may provide an inaccurate picture lacking potentially important nonverbal cues and evaluations of the role of significant others involved in the caller's problem.

Telephone hotlines were first established in the United States and then gradually introduced into Europe, the 'Samaritans' in England being the first in the early 1950s (Varah, 1973). Today in virtually all European countries (both Western and Eastern) such telephone hotlines are in operation 24 hours a day 7 days a week. In Western Europe, they are typically staffed by volunteers and frequently linked to religious bodies. The main problems of callers are interpersonal conflicts and loneliness with an astonishingly low percentage of persons in clear-cut suicidal crises. Real psychiatric emergencies turn up only occasionally. In advertising themselves, these services tend to avoid the term 'psychiatric', and to prefer the term 'friendship' ('telefono amico' in Italy, 'os-amitié' in France, 'Befrienders' by the Samaritans in England). Whether these telephone hotlines prevent suicide or psychiatric hospital admission is uncertain but it seems improbable. They certainly do help callers feel better and facilitate access to other services.

The telephone is also automatically used in many psychiatric emergencies to call in the police or the ambulance, and the way such calls are handled may be decisive for what happens further. Mobile services are as a rule called by 'phone and a skilful emergency worker can already solve a certain proportion of the problems on the 'phone. In the mobile psychiatric emergency service of the Zurich Board of Doctors, one in seven psychiatric emergencies is directly solved by 'phone.

Two more innovative uses of the telephone in psychiatric emergencies deserve mention. In Bratislava (Czechoslovakia) the telephone hotline is manned by nonmedical professionals backed up by 'phone contact with the duty psychiatrist of the mental hospital who may not only counsel the staff but also talk with the client on the 'phone and even arrange admission to a psychiatric hospital. In this way the 'phone helps services not staffed by psychiatrists to quickly get psychiatric advice. General medical emergency hotlines can be similarly backed up by psychiatrists on the 'phone. In the general medical emergency service run by the Vienna Board of Doctors during nights and on weekends, demands for medical help are initiated by 'phone. Since a substantial minority of callers have psychological and psychiatric problems, plans are in train to make a psychiatrist available on the 'phone to directly counsel the doctors or even the callers. A further application of the telephone in psychiatric emergencies is its use by self-help groups of relatives of chronic psychiatric patients for offering informal mutual help and counselling during crisis episodes in the family.

Use of the telephone needs to be extended beyond traditional 'befriending' for less serious problems in order to cover major psychiatric emergencies. In Eastern Europe, telephone hotlines seem to be moving in this direction. There, unlike Western Europe, where volunteers prevail, services are staffed by professionals – psychiatrists, psychologists, social workers and nurses – who usually have their main appointment in a psychiatric institution with 'phone duties as an extra. Thus, the 'phone 'counsellor' has a knowledge of major psychiatric disorders and probably reacts more adequately than volunteers if such conditions are present. In Belgrade, the telephone hotline (Tele-apel) is run by the duty psychiatrist of a psychiatric hospital, and in Ljubljana (Yugoslavia) and Budapest (Hungary) telephone hotlines are respectively sited in a psychiatric hospital and in a psychiatric unit of a general hospital.

The way health care is financed may partly explain why professionals do not more often answer the 'phone in psychiatric emergencies in Western Europe. Where a 'fee for service' operates it is extremely difficult to check payment claims for service if the client stays anonymous and cannot certify that the service has, in fact, been rendered. Staffing by volunteers may be the only viable way to run telephone hotlines. In contrast, in a state health system, as in Eastern Europe, staff may be paid independently of how and where they render the service and the use of professionals for telephone hotlines is easier to organize.

Out-patient services

Direct face-to-face contact conveys a fuller picture of the emergency and offers the chance to do a medical examination, which may lead to more effective intervention. This can be done at the patient's house by a mobile team. When done in outpatients this is on the territory of the clinician. The threshold for using outpatient services depends on their perceived geographical or organizational proximity to a psychiatric unit which may be apparent in the name of the service or its location on the premises of a psychiatric hospital.

The services described here do not dispose of beds but may have access to them. Some crisis or emergency intervention services deliberately renounce beds, taking up the challenge of using natural resources in the community instead of the 'easy' solution of hospitalization. The Crisis Intervention Centre in Vienna is run by a charity but staffed by professionals and had no beds from the very beginning. The Crisis Intervention Service of the Oxford Infirmary started off with beds but soon removed them. These two services seem able to function without beds because they deal mainly with clients in psychosocial crises, and psychiatric emergencies are under-represented.

The proportion of outpatients referred to psychiatric inpatient treatment depends on the types of problems handled by the emergency service. The Centre Psychiatrique d'Orientation et d'Accueil – Psychiatric Centre for Providing Information and Receiving Patients (CPOA) in Paris was founded in 1967 when the psychiatric admission ward of the University Psychiatric Hospital of Sainte Anne was abolished. This outpatient service without direct access to beds serves the whole City of Paris (four million inhabitants) as a central assessment and triage unit. It receives most psychiatric emergencies in Paris which have already made contact with other services (nearly 50% of its patients are sent from outpatient departments of general hospitals), but is also a walk-in clinic (one-quarter of all contacts). The CPOA is increasingly used and the number of attenders was 8,000 in 1967 and has more than doubled since. Two thirds of the patients are referred for inpatient psychiatric treatment to one of the big mental hospitals surrounding Paris. The spectrum of emergencies seen at the CPOA includes severe 'hard core' psychiatric conditions: the largest group are delusional and schizophrenic psychoses (every fourth attender); one in nine patients suffers from chronic alcoholism. The diagnostic spectrum is very similar to the population admitted to psychiatric hospitals. The CPOA is a filter institution which has gained much expertise in the prevention of unnecessary admissions (one-third of attenders are not hospitalized).

Another outpatient service is the 'walk-in-clinic' of the Maudsley Hospital in London (Meng Hooi Lim, 1983). It has a more flexible policy regarding access to beds. While the diagnostic spectrum of attenders is almost identical with that of the CPOA in Paris, only one in eight patients is formally hospitalized. For a period it was possible however – and extensive use was made of this possibility – to 'guest' a patient overnight on a ward of the Maudsley Hospital without officially admitting him. The creation of short-stay wards next door to the emergency rooms of general hospitals in order to prevent psychiatric hospitalization reflects a similar strategy (Kaskey & Ianzito, 1984).

It is thus difficult to run an outpatient service covering the whole spectrum of psychiatric emergencies without having access to beds. Apart from the 'guest-bed' solution in London there is the Yugoslav approach to this problem – the use of day-hospitals. There, explicit use is made of psychiatric day-hospitals to manage psychiatric emergency cases at the 'Mental Health Institute' in Belgrade, which can always be admitted to one of four day-hospitals.

Mobile services

Here, psychiatry is asked to come to the community – a public place or a person's home – outside the usual psychiatric territory. Mobile services are typically asked to intervene less often by the affected individuals themselves than by relatives, friends, other doctors, the police, etc. One reason may be the possible stigmatization of psychiatric emergency intervention in people's homes, where neighbours could become aware of it. Also, mobile services commonly have to deal with patients who are unable or unwilling to contact a service and are more likely to become violent, and to lack insight.

Psychiatric emergency intervention in a person's home can be a make-or-break situation. Skilful intervention offers a unique opportunity for family members to gain decisive insights. On the other hand, having to act under time pressure and the need for a broad range of knowledge – legal, psychopharmacological, techniques of system intervention, etc – may easily overtax the emergency worker, especially if other agencies like the police are also on the scene. A psychiatric emergency team may try to be on the spot before the police arrive to avoid additional complications (Everstine & Everstine, 1983).

The aims of mobile psychiatric emergency services are as manifold as the types of service encountered in Europe. Home visits by team members of sectorized community services for crises of their chronic mental patients aim to prevent hospitalization. A mobile psychiatric emergency service may be called by the police to decide whether to compulsorily admit someone who may have a psychiatric disorder and seems potentially violent to himself or others (in Hamburg, where the mobile emergency service is staffed by a single psychiatrist, 45 out of 143 emergency interventions took place in the home and the remaining 98 at the police station (Kowerk, 1985; Spengler *et al.*, 1983)).

There are different ways of organizing access to a mobile service. The mobile teams of Barnet Psychiatric Hospital in North London and of Hamburg can be called only by other professionals or by the police; in North London these are mainly general practitioners, and in Hamburg they are the general medical emergency service. In contrast, the mobile psychiatric emergency service run by the Zurich Board of Doctors, staffed by a single psychiatrist travelling around in the city in his own car, can be contacted by 'phone even by the general public, but only via a central hotline for all medical emergencies, calls on which are screened by experienced nurses and only then referred to the psychiatrist. Such direct access by the public accounts for roughly half the Zurich calls, the other half of the calls coming from the police or therapeutic institutions. Occasionally (15 % of callers), the patient himself calls in the emergency psychiatrist, and more than one-third of calls are prompted by family members, relatives and other close persons.

Emergency interventions in a person's home provide a fuller picture of the patients' social context and the nature of the emergency. There are, nevertheless, some disadvantages to interventions at home: first the psychiatrist may be rejected if the patient assumes rightly or wrongly that others want to get rid of him. In Zurich, calling the emergency psychiatrist sometimes represents 'delegation' of the problem away from the family to an outside institution (Rothschild, 1982). It needs considerable skill especially in cases of actual or alleged violence or suicidal tendencies to avoid the trap the patient's environment may set for the emergency worker and the patient. Such emergencies can be defused (Everstine & Everstine 1983). Emergency calls come not only from families but also from psychosocial or medical institutions. In the Zurich emergency service, nearly 40% of all interventions end in psychiatric admission. This may be a special problem of an emergency service manned by a single psychiatrist who not only has to act in dangerous situations, but often faces the hard decision of either leaving a problem patient at home or admitting him even when he might do equally well without admission. Emergency *teams* are better off in having more expertise and possibilities of action at their disposal, e.g. one of the team members can remain in the home to ride over the crises when the other team members are called to a fresh emergency elsewhere.

The amount of staff and time available in mobile services seem inversely related to the hospitalization rate. Our observations suggest that mobile services should be generously staffed to relieve pressure on the emergency worker. The first known mobile psychiatric emergency service in the world (Querido, 1968), established in the late 1930s in Amsterdam, used a team approach. In Zurich the psychiatrist is paid by the patient (who is partly reimbursed by social security) and the reimbursement rules do not allow the financing of an additional nonmedical team member. The psychiatrists of the Zurich emergency service went on strike a few years ago to ask for some 'crisis beds' as an intermediate solution.

In conclusion, the emergency worker in mobile services has a complex task. The client may perceive him as an intruder at home and just because of this might not co-operate. A mobile psychiatric emergency service turning up in a person's home can escalate the problem, though, hopefully less so than the escalation caused by the appearance of the police.

Services with overnight stay facilities
In services with overnight stay facilities the client is removed from his own territory to that of the helper. The types of overnight facilities are manifold, as are the reasons for their use. There is large variation in the types of clients, and the treatment methods range from traditional medically oriented psychiatric emergency wards (Reims, Belgrade, Barcelona) to psycho- and sociotherapeutically oriented 'crisis intervention wards' (Munich, West Berlin, Budapest) to informal overnight stay facilities in community mental health centres (Paris and Trieste). Protecting society from violence, preventing suicide, providing relief from a

situation that is unbearable for the patient and/or his family or just providing shelter, are typical goals of such services.

Services with overnight stay facilities have several 'topological' implications. First, the professionals are responsible for the client's well-being while he stays in the service. Second, because more time is available in overnight stay facilities and face-to-face contact is established, assessment and management can be more thorough and efficient. Since the client is under control of the experts, it is fairly easy, if necessary also by using medication, to manage severe problems such as suicidal tendencies, violence or psychotic symptoms. The other 'topological' situation discussed above has disadvantages, either due to lack of face-to-face contact (telephone services) or a lack of time (ambulatory and mobile services). The twin advantages of face-to-face contact and availability of time are, however, accompanied by the disadvantage of an artificial environment which does not allow the fuller assessment of the client's home situation which is possible in mobile services. In some cases, the relief from an overnight stay is only transitory and a lasting solution to the problem is merely postponed. Furthermore, removing a person from his daily living situation may decrease his self-help potential in the community.

Since 1971, when the first 'crisis intervention ward' in Europe was founded in Amsterdam, quite a few such services attracting some publicity were established usually disposing of 10 or 12 (rarely more than 20) beds (Groningen in The Netherlands, Ljubljana in Yugoslavia, Berne in Switzerland, Berlin and Munich in the FRG, and Budapest in Hungary, to mention just a few). Though initially their aims were high, these wards have had rather disappointing experiences. Among the aims of these wards were: prevention of full psychiatric hospitalization, mastery of the patient's problems and discharge within a few days; use of a multidisciplinary team; use of the crisis to aid personality growth. Few of these aims could be fulfilled. The constant pressure to admit new clients, impossibility of clearing up all problems within a few days and the lack of aftercare facilities, often leads to psychiatric hospitalization. Most of these wards admit selectively, refusing overtly suicidal and aggressive patients and those with severe alcohol problems or psychotic symptoms, partly to avoid psychiatric stigma that would decrease the acceptability of the service by people in mainly psychosocial crises.

Specialized/centralized versus comprehensive/decentralized services

The value of specialized and centralized services for emergency psychiatry and crisis intervention is questioned by the recent development of sectorized community psychiatric services in several European countries. These sectorized services – which are very differently organized in different countries and whose detailed discussion is beyond the scope of this paper – tend to claim that they, not the specialized services, should be the providers of emergency psychiatric care.

In France, the Ministry of Health sent out a circular in 1979 requesting efforts to establish a 24-hour psychiatric emergency service in all sectors. Progress in establishing sectorized emergency care has, however, been very slow. A rare exception where a sectorized service provides a 24-hour 7-day-a-week emergency care is psychiatric sector 5 (Santé Mentale 5 – SM5) covering the sixth *arrondissement* in Paris (with about 30,000 inhabitants). Psychiatric sector 5 has a comprehensive community mental health centre in a large office building in its centre offering outpatient care, home visits and three beds for overnight stay. It also has 40 beds in the nearby psychiatric hospital of Sainte Anne. All services are under one and the same medical directorship. The centre is generously staffed with nurses, doctors and psychologists, who wear casual clothes, create an informal atmosphere and seem enthusiastic in their work. Of the 524 clients asking for help in 1983 (50% of whom were new cases) a large proportion were long-term users. We were told that only 50% of the new cases had a real psychiatric problem, the others having 'social problems', asking for psychotherapy, etc. In 1982, 144 clients spent a total of 844 nights at the centre. The advantage of such a comprehensive service is its continuity of care, as patients seen in crisis or an emergency are offered after-care by the same team of professionals. There is a latent rivalry between this decentralized comprehensive service and the centralized specialized emergency service (CPOA) for the whole city of Paris and its environs described earlier. However, there is some co-operation; in 1982 every sixth referral to the community mental health centre came from the CPOA.

We have described this Parisian situation in detail since there are indications that in other parts of Europe the establishment of comprehensive community psychiatric services can jeopardize existing specialized crisis intervention and emergency services. Amsterdam, with the oldest mobile service for psychiatric emergencies and the first European crisis intervention ward (established in 1971), emergency psychiatry and crisis intervention has been decentralized and is carried out as one of many tasks by five community mental health centres working around the clock.

In a sense, comprehensiveness versus specialization in the psychiatric care system in Europe has come full circle. Traditional hospital-based psychiatric services were 'comprehensive' in that they were the only services available and had to fulfil all tasks, including emergency care. One reason for the springing up of new specialized services – not only emergency and crisis services but also rehabilitation services – was the recognition of the deficiencies of the traditional psychiatric hospital located far away from the community. Nowadays, as sectorized community psychiatric services are increasingly established, the role of these specialized services is being questioned. What are the tradeoffs of specialized and centralized services versus comprehensive and decentralized services? Desirable as 24-hours, 7-days-a-week sectorized comprehensive psychiatric services might be, several obstacles impede their implementation. First, such services are very costly. Wherever attempts were made to establish such a service, planners have not got far. In France, the psychiatric sector 5 in Paris is still one of very few examples. In Trieste, Italy economic limitations forced planners to close decentralized community mental health centres at night and to establish a centralized emergency service. A second limit to the capability of comprehensive sectorized community psychiatric services taking over responsibility for emergencies and crises, is the infrequent occurrence of emergencies in a small sector. In Southern European countries, sector size ranges from 30,000 to 80,000 inhabitants. Good handling of emergencies is a complex task which cannot be learned from books alone, so the opportunity to gain experience is crucial, yet limited if emergencies are rare. In psychiatric sector 5 of Paris an average of one emergency occurs in 24 hours; given that different team members are on duty at different times, a long period has to elapse before an individual staff member gains much experience in handling psychiatric emergencies. In contrast, in a busy centralized emergency service, such as the CPOA, staff members quickly acquire extensive experience and are ideally suited to carry out postgraduate training in the field.

Comprehensive community psychiatric services have several advantages, the most important being the possibility of continuity of care. For chronic psychiatric patients living in the community who develop a crisis, the chance is high that they and their social field are already known to the staff member on duty, either personally or from team discussions. The staff member would thus better understand, say, a family conflict in which the buck is being passed on to an institution. In contrast, a centralized specialized service covering a large area allows less detailed knowledge about particular patients, although that service will also have its 'chronic users' and 'repeaters'. Comprehensive sectorized community services also offer follow-up care which is usually not possible from a busy centralized and specialized emergency service. Maintaining contact with a patient with whom an intensive relationship has been built up during an emergency is more satisfying than losing sight of him once the emergency intervention is over, as is usual in a busy centralized service. Specialized emergency service staff complain that this lack of follow-up, of feedback, contributes to their burn-out which is also nourished by other factors like the frequent confrontation with violence, need to decide about compulsory admission, lack of information when deciding about treatment decisions, etc. Further advantages of integrating emergency care and crisis intervention into comprehensive psychiatric services are the availability of the skills of a multiprofessional team, less of the time pressure characteristic of centralized specialized services with high case-loads and the readiness of team members to go into the community.

An intermediate solution to the centralized/specialized versus comprehensive/decentralized dilemma has been found in Trieste. There, a catchment area of approximately 280,000 inhabitants is served by seven community mental health centres which, among many other functions, also accept psychiatric emergencies by day. Patients arriving before 8pm may also stay overnight if needed. At night, however, these community mental health centres do not accept clients and psychiatric emergencies are dealt with by a centralized 8-bed psychiatric unit at the general hospital, which also offers psychiatric consultation to the general emergency room. This model is unique in its intense links between the decentralized community mental health centres and the centralized emergency room in the general hospital, since both services are run by the same staff. Doctors working in the decentralized community mental health centres during normal working hours are on duty at the centralized psychiatric emergency service several nights a month. Thus, each of them knows intimately how both services function. Co-operation between the two services is nearly perfect. Patients who are admitted to the centralized psychiatric emergency service are soon collected by staff from the decentralized community mental health centre who immediately take care of them. Beds are therefore often empty, especially during daytime. The system in Trieste seems to work smoothly. It not only prevents escalation of emergencies but probably also prevents development of many emergencies themselves through the continuous work of the community mental health centres and their easy accessibility during normal working hours. The Trieste system, however, is probably more suitable for the socially underprivileged and for chronic mental patients living in the community than for neurotic depressives and suicidal patients.

Conclusion

While a consensus seems to be emerging in Europe about how rehabilitation services for psychiatric patients should look, we are still far from knowing the best way to provide psychiatric emergency care and crisis intervention. Attempts at establishing specialized services for this purpose over the last 15 years have been supplanted by a trend to set up comprehensive community services which, *inter alia*, provide emergency care and crisis intervention. Moreover, some countries are now trying to reintegrate psychiatric emergency care into the general medical care system.

While we are still searching for guidelines about how to organize emergency and crisis intervention services, it is also evident that immense financial, legal and administrative barriers stand in the face of implementing new solutions. As long as we professionals do not know what we really want, politicians and administrators will not be able or willing to adapt legislation and budgets. We lack proper evaluation of new models of psychiatric emergency care and crisis intervention. Such evaluations prove to be extremely difficult, given the specific work conditions in emergency services and the pressures on staff.

References

Bassuk, E. L. (1985). Psychiatric emergency services: Can they cope as last-resort facilities? In (Lipton, R. R. & Goldfinger, S. M., eds) *Emergency Psychiatry at the Crossroads*. pp. 11–20, Jossey-Bass Inc., San Francisco, London.

Bassuk, E. & Gerson, S. (1980). Chronic crisis patients: A discrete Clinical Group. *Am. Journal of Psychiatry*, **137**, 1513–17.

Caroli, F. & Olié, J. P. (1979). Nouvelles formes déséquilibre mental. *Congrés de psychiatrie et de neurologie de langue française*, Angers Masson, Paris.

Cooper, J. E. (1979). Crisis admission units and emergency psychiatric services. *Public Health in Europe*, **11**, Regional Office for Europe, World Health Organization, Copenhagen.

Everstine, D. S. & Everstine, L. E. (1983). *People in Crisis: Strategic Therapeutic Interventions*. Brunner/Mazel, New York.

Groves, J. (1978). Taking care of the hateful patient. *New England Journal of Medicine*, **298**, 883–7.

Häfner-Ranabauer, W. & Günzler, G. (1984). Entwicklung und Funktion des psychiatrischen Krisen- und Notfalldienstes in Mannheim. *Fortschritte der Neurologie Psychiatrie*, **52**, 83–90.

Kaskey, G. B. & Ianzito, B. M. (1984). Development of an emergency psychiatric treatment unit. *Hospital Community Psychiatry*, **35**, 1220–2.

Katschnig, H. & Cooper, J. (1988). Emergency psychiatry and crisis intervention. In (Freeman, H. & Bennett, D. eds.) *Handbook of Community Psychiatry*. Churchill Livingstone, Chichester.

Katschnig, H., Konieczna, T. & Cooper, J. (eds) (In Press). *Crisis Intervention and Emergency Psychiatric Services in Europe*. World Health Organization, Copenhagen.

Katschnig, H. & Konieczna, T. (In Press). Report on a study of crisis intervention units and psychiatric emergency services in Europe, part 2: City reports. In (Katschnig, H., Konieczna, T. & Cooper, J. eds.) *Crisis Intervention and Emergency Psychiatric Services in Europe*. World Health Organization, Copenhagen.

Klerman, G. L. (1985). Community mental health developments in the USA. In (Rapport, R. N. ed.) *Research and Action, a Collaborative Interactive Approach*. Cambridge University Press, Cambridge.

Kowerk, H. (1985). Die ärztliche Entscheidungssituation bei Zwangseinweisungen. *Recht & Psychiatrie* **3**, 138–49.

Meng Hooi Lim (1983). A psychiatric emergency clinic: A study of attendances over six months. *British Journal of Psychiatry*, **143**, 460–6.

Pisarcik, G. (1982). Interagency and intraagency collaboration. In Gorton, J. G. & Partridge, R. eds.) *Practice and Management of Psychiatric Emergency Care*. pp. 392–405, C. V. Mosby, St. Louis.

Querido, A. (1968). The shaping of community mental health care. *British Journal of Psychiatry*, **114**, 293–301.

Ratna, L. (1982). Crisis intervention in psychogeriatrics: A two-year follow-up study. *British Journal of Psychiatry*, **141**, 296–301.

Rothschild, B. (1982). Achtung: *Psychiater*, Beltz, Weinheim, Basel.

Segal, S. P., Watson, M. A. & Scott Nelson, L. (1985). Equity in the application of civil commitment criteria. In (Lipton, F. R. & Goldfinger, S. M. eds) *Emergency Psychiatry at the Crossroads*. pp. 93–105, Jossey-Bass, San Francisco, London.

Spengler, A., Hagenah, R. & Friedrich, G. (1983). Behandlungsindikationen bei psychiatrischen Notfallen. *Psychiatrische Praxis* **10**, 200–8.

Varah, C. (1973). *The Samaritans in the '70s. To Befriend the Suicidal and Despairing*. Constable, London.

Walker, J. I. (1983). *Psychiatric Emergencies. Intervention and Resolution*. J. P. Lippincott, Philadelphia, London.

8

Emergency care for the acute and severely mentally ill

Steven P. Segal

Psychiatric emergency contacts throughout the world generally involve: 1. the presence of an urgent situation defying usual patterns of coping, 2. the failure of one's social network to circumscribe or to ameliorate the crisis and 3. convenient access to the emergency service. These contacts can be conceived of as complex interactions between the person and his/her environment which generally fall into one of two categories: 1. They are life-threatening emergencies – involving violence to self and/or others or a deteriorated pattern of functioning giving rise to an imminent concern for the individual's capacity to assume responsibility for his/her self-protection and well-being. 2. They are crises resulting from 'life transitions, traumatic experiences, maturational/developmental stages, psychopathological decompensation, existential despair, and even routine problems in daily living' (Birk & Bassuk, 1984, p. 3).

The life-threatening problems are often referred to as 'real' (cf. Katschnig & Konieczna, Chap. 7) or 'genuine' psychiatric emergencies by mental health professionals because they require immediate symptom containment and often result in civil commitment. Unfortunately, not enough is known about the nature of the relationship between the 'real' emergencies and the second group of crisis situations. For example, we do not know the extent to which these two types of emergencies are categorically different phenomena or exist on a continuum such that failure to act in a less serious situation – one we would place in the crisis category – may lead to having to act in a situation that looks more like a 'real' life-threatening emergency.

Katschnig & Konieczna's comprehensive discussion of psychiatric emergency services in Europe, in Chapter 7 of this book, has made my task relatively easy.

Their paper revolves around three issues: first, the classification of emergency services; second, the description of types of patients in need of such services; third, a discussion of the advantages and disadvantages of specialized, centralized service models on the one hand, versus comprehensive, decentralized service models on the other.

Psychiatric emergency services in the United States have developed largely under the impetus of the 1963 Community Mental Health Centers and Facility Act which made 24-hour emergency service one of the required services of a community mental health centre. As was true of all services required in the community mental health centres legislation, the focus of service effort was a preventative public health approach, assuming a continuum between crisis care and the provision of genuine psychiatric emergency care. The full spectrum of psychiatric emergency services described by Katschnig & Konieczna in Europe was developed in the United States in the early 1960s; this included telephone-based services, outpatient-based services, mobile type services – under the rubric of psychiatric emergency teams (PET) and/or 'flying squads' – and services located in general hospitals offering the opportunity for overnight stays.

In developing a classification of psychiatric services, Katschnig & Konieczna use a descriptive concept based upon what they call a 'psychosocial topology' related primarily to the power relationship between the patient and the facility. In particular, they have noted some of the expanded potential of the telephone service in dealing with serious problems and have emphasized the power the patient has in controlling his or her own participation in the service when it is conducted over the telephone. In the United States many commentators have viewed those people using telephone emergency services as differing in character from those people coming to emergency rooms in general hospitals to receive services. Those using telephone services tend to present situations similar to those described as 'crisis situations' as opposed to the 'life-threatening' emergencies which are more likely to appear in emergency rooms or could be the focus of mobile emergency services.

In the United States, there exists no unique organization of emergency care. Well-integrated emergency care systems are rare and have become rarer since the demise of the community mental health centres legislation which offered communities a financial incentive to maintain a fully integrated system of care. Today, communities in the United States rely primarily on the general hospital psychiatric emergency room or the general hospital emergency room augmented by psychiatric services to deal with increasing numbers of crises and life-threatening psychiatric emergencies. To some extent, the increase in the utilization of general hospital psychiatric emergency rooms is due to the decreasing availability of community care for the seriously mentally ill in the United States and to the general abandonment of state responsibility for the long-term care and treatment of this population. Consequently, large numbers of seriously and chronically mentally ill adults receive services in psychiatric emergency rooms only when they have deteriorated into a crisis state.

In the provision of emergency services in the United States, the psychosocial topology approach of Katschnig & Konieczna complements the social role or social work approach offered by Kadushin, (1968). The latter approach describes services as supportive, supplemental, or substitutive of current roles in terms of their potential for managing both life-threatening and nonlife-threatening problems.

In the management of life-threatening situations, it is particularly important to address the physical, legal, pharmacological, psychological and social needs of the patient. *Supportive* services are those services involving the least interference with an individual's ongoing social roles. They consist of crisis intervention types of services which enable people to cope with problematic situations by themselves, using their own resources. These services can be delivered by trained personnel over the telephone, by mobile mental health units, or by outpatient practitioners as well as by staff in the context of the emergency room. They help the individual put the crisis situation in perspective and help with assessment of available resources. In many respects, these services help modify two of the three major considerations for being in the service in the first place; these involve the individual's perception that the social network has failed to support him/her in a crisis or that he/she fails to possess the coping skills necessary to alleviate the crisis. Often such services are delivered in the form of counselling, whether it be legal, health care, psychological or social needs that are addressed in the individual's failure to cope.

Supplemental services are those additional aids or resources necessary to enable people to maintain their life situations. One program not mentioned by Katschnig & Konieczna is a 'neighbourhood watch' program. This emergency service functions as a warning device to reduce the seriousness of emergencies experienced by people. For example, upon developing a major depressive episode, one psychotic patient of my acquaintance discontinues his eating. Routinely, he receives subsidized meals in a local restaurant. The restaurateur may notice the patient's absence at such meals and may express concern about the patient to the patient's case manager who will drop in to visit the patient on an informal basis just to see how he is doing.

Substitutive care, on the other hand, provides a place where an individual can withdraw from the pressures of his/her normal social role. Facilities providing such care are usually inpatient, overnight facilities including emergency services units in general hospitals. They may also include day hospitals, community mental health centres with beds (as used in Trieste, Italy), and nonhospital, subacute crisis houses. In these facilities, people are removed from the stress of their roles to stabilize and to establish a new equilibrium enabling them to return to their environment.

The second issue addressed by Katschnig & Konieczna relates to the type of people who need emergency services. They distinguish three types of patients: those in acute psychosocial crisis, patients with acute psychiatric conditions needing urgent medical attention, and chronic psychiatric patients living in the community. This typology provides a fine description of the types of people we see in emergency rooms or in crisis services. However, a greater elaboration on this typology might link it to the classification of services which would be most appropriate to each patient's needs in the emergency care process. Generally, individuals in acute psychosocial crises tend to avail themselves of, or be in need of, supportive services to help them work through their crises. Patients with acute psychiatric conditions needing urgent medical attention tend to use supplemental and substitutive services to cope with their crises. Finally, chronic psychiatric patients living in the community tend to avail themselves of the full range of supportive, supplemental and substitutive services depending upon the availability of well-planned community support system services in their communities.

A crucial component of the emergency assessment in determining the level of care and answering the question of who needs psychiatric emergency care is not addressed by Katschnig & Konieczna; this involves the degree of dangerousness associated with the patient's presentation of self and circumstances. My research group has been able to describe reliably the assessment of perceived dangerousness of patients coming to emergency rooms and would see this component of the assessment as a key factor in determining the need for more substitutive as opposed to supportive or supplemental services (Segal, Watson, & Nelson, 1986).

In addressing the issue of providing the appropriate level of psychiatric emergency care, the reliability of the assessment of the patient's current condition seems crucial. High reliability of assessment can be achieved in two areas: the assessment of acute physiological crisis, and the assessment of perceived dangerousness. While the validity of the latter remains in question, the principles of equity and least restrictive alternative treatment are best protected by using these two assessments in matching a person's needs to the types of services available. The principle of equity in this context refers to a patient's right to have equal access to assessment and treatment recognized as meeting minimum practice standards. Access to assessment and treatment conforming to minimum practice standards should not be impeded by context factors which lead to discrimination against one group or another. For example, being unfortunate enough to have one's assessment done at a time when the service is overcrowded might make it impossible to receive an adequate assessment. The latter results from inappropriate knowledge of or concern with the impact of staff/patient ratios on quality of care (Segal, Watson, & Nelson, 1986). It can be ameliorated or prevented by having additional 'on-call' staff or by diversion plans. These strategies will redirect incoming patients to less crowded facilities.

The third issue discussed by Katschnig & Konieczna is a planning issue which in many respects resolves itself in the nature of the geographic area being served: specialized centralized services versus decentralized, comprehensive services. It would certainly be most desirable to have comprehensive, decentralized services and to resolve the issue of practitioner competence by rotating staff to high-risk areas where appropriate experience can be obtained. Specialized centralized services clearly move people away from the environment we wish them to stay with. These services are sometimes more cost-effective in the short run. However, given the experience of the mental hospital, there is some question of their effectiveness over the long haul, i.e. they are prone to become substitutive types of facilities rather than supportive or supplemental care systems and to inappropriately retain people for long periods of time, placing them at high risk of iatrogenic effects. Kiesler (1982) summarizes the results of over 20 clinical trials indicating that all well-planned alternatives to hospital treatment prove themselves to be more effective than hospital treatment in situations requiring any type of substitutive care other than physiological intervention.

A central disagreement with Katschnig & Konieczna's presentation of the European situation revolves around their description of the specialized, centralized Servizi di Diagnosi e Cura (SDC), the general hospital inpatient ward in Trieste, Italy. Based upon my experience in Trieste, it is my understanding that discussion among the psychiatric consultants and their primario has been focussed on a debate over whether or not to close this unit totally. The psychiatrists staffing the unit think that they can get along without it. The mental health centres have beds which can be opened as needed and staffed only when they are used. The SDC beds are in no way seen as a substitute for the community mental health centre beds. The debate over the use of the mental health services in Trieste points to the true third issue in the provision of psychiatric emergency services. This involves the mission of the service with regard to how the service views the provision of psychiatric emergency care.

The service's mission refers to the goal or function that the emergency room believes it fulfils in the process of delivering services. It is this mission which will determine how staff relate to their clientele. The Trieste SDC is a unit of eight beds which has as its mission the goal of keeping those beds empty. Of all such facilities I saw in Italy, this was the only facility in which the beds actually were empty. There, psychiatrists were able to provide supportive or supplemental types of services, in most cases in lieu of substitutive services, to meet the needs of the populace of Trieste. The staff did use the beds when it was necessary to use them, but the beds were definitely underused. As noted by Katschnig & Konieczna, the use of substitutive care – the hospital bed – is the expedient and unfortunate solution. Utilization of such services is inappropriate because of the high probability of iatrogenic effects associated with hospitalization as well as the unwarranted expense of hospitalization when in fact an alternative mode of care under most circumstances is more appropriate (Kiesler, 1982). Such alternatives may be substitutive of total roles, as is the case with the use of crisis houses in the United States. These facilities often do not retain the stigma associated with the hospital and do enable the patient to cope with his or her crisis situation in a more normalized environment.

The use of the hospital is an easy solution to substitutive care – as noted by Katschnig & Konieczna – because to some extent it is very much a part of the training of psychiatrists. In England, I observed a mental health service that had functioned very effectively for ten years with one ward. Yet, with the addition of a new consultant who worked from a traditional hospital perspective, in the course of one year this service had managed to fill two additional wards that were assigned to it. There was no increase in the incidence of disorder observed in this community. This occurrence seems to reflect a preference for psychiatric practice in the context of ward-based care.

It is my observation that the situation in which the particular mission of an emergency room influences the patient selection process occurs with perhaps the same frequency as the situation in which patient need determines the mission. Some emergency rooms view themselves as centres for crisis intervention where they evaluate and treat both life-threatening and nonlife-threatening emergencies. Over time they come to serve both types of patients. Other emergency services view themselves as dealing only with life-threatening emergencies in an evaluative format and, thus, restrict their service population. In the latter case, the goal of the room is to determine whether or not the emergency is truly a life-threatening situation and to make the appropriate admission to an inpatient ward in a general hospital or the referral to a crisis facility. One director of a facility that emphasizes an evaluative format as opposed to a crisis intervention format in life-threatening situations eliminated all his social work staff. He argued that they were spending too much time discussing the family and the context in which the person had his/her problems, and, in this respect, the services were not cost effective. Thus, currently in this room, when individuals who are chronically mentally ill arrive at the beginning of the month in an acute psychotic crisis largely because they have failed to get their welfare checks, the emergency staff evaluates their degree of psychiatric disturbance, misses the context of the crisis, treats patients with medications, and moves them on to an inpatient facility. Similarly, without the input of medical staff there is a danger that organicity will be overlooked in the emergency room. Therefore, in dealing with psychiatric emergencies, it is most important to address not only the types of people in need of service and the types of services available to meet their needs but to define very clearly the mission of psychiatric emergency care. This mission should be that of promoting least restrictive care by providing whatever supportive, supplemental, and, if necessary, substitutive care is needed to enable people to return to a state of equilibrium which enables them to function best in their current community environments.

Acknowledgements

Special thanks belong to all my colleagues in England and Italy for their co-operation and support. The research was supported by the Center for International Exchange of Scholars, Western European Regional Research Fulbright Award; NIMH, Grant No. MH37310. The opinions expressed herein are those of the author, not the funding organizations.

References

Birk, A. W., & Bassuk, E. L. (1984). The concept of emergency care. In (E. L. Bassuk, & A. W. Birk, eds), *Emergency psychiatry* (pp. 3–18). Plenum, New York.

Kadushin, A. (1968). *Child Welfare Services*. Macmillan, New York.

Katschnig, H. & Konieczna, T. (1990). Innovations in delivery of emergency services. In (I. M. Marks & R. Scott, eds), *Innovations in Mental Health Care Delivery*, Chapter 7. Cambridge University Press, Cambridge.

Kiesler, C. A. (1982). Mental hospitals and alternative care: Noinstitutionalization as potential public policy for mental patients. *American Psychologist*, **37(4)**, 349–61.

Segal, S. P., Watson, M. A. & Nelson, L. S. (1986). Indexing civil commitment in psychiatric emergency rooms. *Annals of the American Academy of Political and Social Science*, **484**, 56–69.

Part II

IMPEDIMENTS

Section D: Sociopolitical

Commentary by editors and John Carrier

Part II of this book discusses why apparently successful demonstration projects may fail to disseminate widely through the care system. Some lack of receptivity is due to sociopolitical, administrative, economic and professional factors. Knowledge of these factors is at present very sketchy, but some of the relevant issues are suggested in the rest of this book.

If helpful innovations are to spread through a mental health care delivery system they must surmount sociopolitical barriers. Inevitably health care systems are a patchwork of compromises in a constraining social field. Rudolf Klein (1983) has written that

> if the politics of the NHS over the past thirty-five years demonstrate anything,
> it is that there is no way of reconciling all the various interests, all the various
> competing policy aims and values that are inevitably and inextricably involved
> in the health care policy arena ... from this perspective the NHS is an institution
> which internalises and reflects tensions and conflicts inevitable in a pluralistic
> society[1]

Klein suggests that the NHS represents a victory of tactical considerations over administrative logic and coherence. In a sense that is true for all systems, and indeed has been true for all organisms throughout evolution.

In Section D, Carrier and Marmor deal with the issue in the United Kingdom and in the United States. For both countries health care expenditure is a major item, although the United Kingdom percentage of Gross National Product spent on health services is still about half that spent in the United States. To put it in perspective, however, Carrier points out that in the United Kingdom, for 1988/9 the forecast for taxes raised by the sale of tobacco products and of spirits, beer and wine, was a yield of £5 billion and £4·5 billion respectively, whilst the expenditure on health and personal social services in the United Kingdom for 1988/89 was forecast at £20·7 billion.[2] In other words, the taxes from alcohol and tobacco sales raise almost half the total expenditure on health and personal social services.

We could add that, while the successful United Kingdom pharmaceutical industry spends fully one-sixth of its turnover on research and advertising, less than 1% of the United Kingdom total health care expenditure is on relevant research and dissemination of its findings. These are sobering pointers to priorities. The political emphasis in both countries on cost constraints has thwarted mental health care developments in this decade.

Though the current rhetoric is of scarcity, in fact society's actual resources are now far more abundant than they have ever been historically. With relatively fewer people, we produce more food, goods and services than ever before.

The issue concerns priorities. Household expenditure in the United Kingdom on food in 1986 (at 1985 prices) was £31 billion. Consumer expenditure on beer and other alcoholic drinks amounted to £16 billion, or roughly half that spent on food. If we add to that the £6 billion spent on tobacco, then together the spending on these two health-damaging products is two-thirds of that spent on food.[3]

A mere 3% of people working in agriculture produces a hefty surplus of food, greater than 90% of the population working on the land did centuries ago. The same huge rise in relative and absolute productivity is seen in the manufacture of goods. Much of the population is thus released to work in other sectors — education, transport, media, entertainment, tourism, and of course, health care. All these sectors jostle for manpower and money, and health care often loses out, mental health care perhaps most of all.

The total Gross Current Expenditure on Mental Illness in patient services in the United Kingdom in 1985/86 was £1 billion; and for mental illness outpatient services was £72 million. This amounts to 11% of the total spending on hospital and community health services, although psychiatric beds still formed 36% of all hospital beds in 1985.[4] Even so, in 1986, hospital beds occupied by mentally ill people fell by a further 5%, and outpatient attendances rose by 0·8% with psychiatric day-patient attendances rising by 2·7% A Department of Health memorandum to the House of Commons Social Services Committee informs us that 'between March 1986 and March 1987 the number of residents supported by personal social service departments in the United Kingdom fell by a further 6·1%'. The view of the Department of Health that this fall 'reflects greater availability of social security support for people in voluntary and private homes'[5] may be over-optimistic, premature and not borne out by workers in the field.

Today's zero sum game is nothing new, but it is played more openly. The building of the nineteenth century mental hospitals meant that other worthy causes went short. Funds have always been competed for by different client groups, by the mentally ill versus the mentally handicapped, by the physically ill against the blind and the deaf. Current resources may be more abundant than in the past but they remain and always will be finite, and competing claims on them are, and always will be, greater than ever as expectations rise.

We are parsimonious today compared to some of our predecessors. The lavish building of many large mental hospitals by our nineteenth century forebears represented the largest nonmilitary expenditure until that time (John Stillwell, personal communication). With the wisdom of hindsight we might question the policy on which that money was spent. But the willingness to spend on the mentally ill was there. Though today we are much wealthier than a century ago, we are less ready to fund mental health care. The proportion of the GNP spent on mental health has gone down, not up, in one of the world's fastest expanding economies – South Korea (Norman Sartorius, personal communication). We spend a lot of time formulating policy but little in testing it and still less in disseminating the results of the research.

The United States is more decentralized than the United Kingdom, making co-ordinated problem-solving more difficult. On the other hand, pluralism facilitates informed comparison of how different policies work at different sites. Marmor indicates that what works is not so much persuasion as pork barrel politics, which concentrate the benefits on a small group while diffusing the costs across other groups, e.g. the funding of a local facility out of general funds. A complementary trend is bile barrel politics, where the loss is concentrated on one group and the benefits are diffused across other groups, e.g. the dumping of mental patients from a wide area into a single hospital.

The mentally ill make up a substantial minority of the growing army of the homeless. A major cause of homelessness is not only deinstitutionalization but also urban renewal and rising house prices. In the United States there are Federal moves to help the housing of the mentally ill by funding the difference between the cost of their housing and what they can afford on social security. This funding difference has become a major issue in the United Kingdom coinciding with a dramatic change in the administration of social security benefits, the decline in the number of average daily occupied mental illness beds, and the decline in public expenditure on housing. The increase in the social security budget from 17% of United Kingdom public expenditure in 1950 to 33% in 1986 reflected a rise in the elderly pensionable population.[6] The number of psychiatric beds declined from 193,000 in 1959 to 108,000 in 1985.[7] Over the same period the number of psychiatric hospitals in England actually increased from 303 to 492, due to the demise of the 2,000 bed hospital in the early 1970s and a corresponding rise in the number of small hospitals.[8]

A worrying trend is the decline in public expenditure on housing. Few discharged mentally ill people have the buying power to compete in the private housing market. The proportion of public expenditure on housing declined from 9·6% in 1979 to 4·3% by 1986. In real terms the decline was from £5·4 billion in 1981/82 to £3·5 billion in 1987/88 with plans for £3·8 billion in 1988/89.[9] Given the central importance of publicly provided housing for this client group, the omens are not propitious for community care in the United Kingdom.

The British Griffiths Report 'Community Care: Agenda for Action',[10] was published in 1988. Griffiths' philosophy was that 'no person should be discharged without a clear package of care devised and without being the responsibility of a named care worker'. He recommended that a Minister should be 'clearly and publicly identified as responsible for community care', that 'the primary responsibility for Community Care should correctly lie with the Local Authority' (personal social services, not the health authority) and that 'there must be a clear framework within which local and health authorities are working out their own process of coordination' The United Kingdom Government had not formally commented on this Griffiths' proposal for Community Care 15 months after its publication. This presumably reflects the Government's reluctance to give more responsibility to local authorities whose powers it has considerably whittled away in the last few years. Instead, the Government considered the 'funding crisis' in the NHS and published a White Paper 'Working for Patients'[11] in 1989. If it is implemented it will fundamentally alter the manner in which the NHS works. Opposition from professionals is strong. Services for mentally ill people again look likely to be relegated to the back burner by concerns over the future delivery of all health services in the United Kingdom. Whether President Bush's speech to Congress in February 1989 augurs better for clients of the mental health services in the United States remains to be seen.

Finally, in Chapter 11 in this section, Dr Sartorius deals with a different set of sociopolitical obstacles to mental health care delivery. They are rarely written about but no less important for that. The obstacles are analysed across European countries but are applicable more generally.

Dr Sartorius shows how few reliable and agreed indicators are available on which to compare the mental health service systems of different countries. Even when indicators appear to be similar their meaning may differ substantially from one country to another and there can be considerable regional differences within countries.

Despite such problems, however, some European trends are apparent. On the whole, European countries for which data are available have a broadly similar pattern of services; the number of large mental hospitals has fallen and of psychiatric units in general hospitals has risen. European psychiatric services have tended to become decentralized. Cost constraints and an emphasis on quality assurance have become salient. Concern about confidentiality has led to the termination of several psychiatric case registers. Interprofessional rivalries have sharpened, and lack of co-ordination among various mental health sectors has continued.

On certain indicators European countries differ vastly – fully 80-fold on number of nurses per psychiatrist, nine-fold on numbers of admissions per psychiatric bed and of outpatient contacts, and five-fold on number of psychiatrists. Understanding the reasons for such differences and the effects of those differences on mental health care delivery could lead to more effective ways of improving the quality of services.

Notes

1. Klein, R. (1983). *The Politics of the National Health Service*. Chapter 6, p. 193. Longman, England.
2. Financial Statement and Budget Report 1988–89. HMSO March 1988. House of Commons paper no. 361.
3. United Kingdom National Accounts. Central Statistical Office. Table 4.5, p. 41. 'Personal Sector Consumers' expenditure classified by Commodity at current prices.' HMSO, London, 1988.
4. Programme Budget. Hospital and Community Health Services. House of Commons Session 1987/88. Social Services Committee. Public Expenditure on the Social Services. House of Commons paper 548. Page 23. Table 3.1.
5. Programme Budget. Hospital and Community Health Services. House of Commons Session 1987/88. Social Services Committee. Public Expenditure on the Social Services. House of Commons paper 548, p. 33.
6. *Compendium of Health Statistics*. Office of Health Economics, 6th edition 1987. London. Table 2.10, p. 35.
7. *Compendium of Health Statistics*. Office of Health Economics, 6th edition 1987. London. Table 3.9, p. 20.
8. *Health and Personal Social Service Statistics for England*. 1987 edition. DHSS London.
9. UK: The Government's Expenditure Plans. Cm.288. HM Treasury 1988.
10. Sir Roy Griffiths (1988). *Community Care, Agenda for Action*. HMSO, London.
11. The Health Service (1989). *Working for Patients*. HMSO, London.

9

Sociopolitical influences on mental health care policy in the United Kingdom

John Carrier

In this paper, a broad approach to the discussion of the political and economic context of mental health care is used. It is difficult to separate the recent political history of the NHS from the economics and finance of the service, as well as from its administration, organisation and planning. For the purpose of this paper, they will be treated as analytically distinct but will be brought together to show their influence on the mental health services in the United Kingdom.

Despite the significance of 'Thatcherism' in the years 1979–90, the notion of 'influence' goes beyond the impact of modern party politics on health care and has as much to do with the relationship between central government and local authorities, and especially decision-making by local health authorities. A publication (Holmes, 1986) referred to 'Mrs Thatcher's defiant ideological style as having replaced the pragmatism of the 1945–75 era', reversing the 'socialist ratchet effect'. This reversal, it is argued, has jettisoned a long list of state controls, especially those concerned with an incomes policy and the abandonment of target growth rates. At the same time inflation has been brought under control, the Trade Unions 'tamed', and the drift towards 'corporatism' halted.

Economic issues

Two major problems have remained intractable since 1979: the increase in unemployment and the control of public expenditure. The first of these now seems to be endemic, perhaps the price paid for a lower inflation rate, but with a serious effect on the second. The United Kingdom Government has made 'across the board' public spending cuts. The main targets for 'cuts' have been the social services, education, local government finance, housing and the Civil Service. Health 'cuts' have been difficult to implement due to the high degree of public support for the Service, the fact that it is the country's largest employer (of highly unionized labour) and the Government's commitment to redistribution of resources within the services.

Policy implementation

Any attempt to implement progressive social policies on behalf of a dependent client group requires special conditions if these policies are to move from normative approach to practical outcome. Hall *et al.* (1975) suggest that such policies need to be feasible in the eyes of professionals and administrators, to be legitimate in the eyes of legislators and the public (consumers and taxpayers) and to have the support of partisans whose commitment will see such policies through from chrysalis to butterfly. The pressure group activity which often accompanies such progressive movements, and is usually the dynamic force behind them, also requires individual supporters with the capacity, opportunity, motivation and commitment to their cause.

To implement mental health policies which involve the closing down of large nineteenth-century mental hospitals, decommissioning old buildings and providing a new service requires a propitious political and economic climate. The political climate needs to be an enabling one, with general unanimity about the values of integration, community, other-directedness and altruism. The ideal economic context would be one in which growth would be steady and sustained, competition for public resources would not be seen as a burden on the economy and some version of Keynesianism rather than monetarism would be the overriding theoretical framework underpinning economic debates and activities. Relationships between central and local government would need to be mutual, respectful and symbiotic. For the United Kingdom none of these ideal conditions have existed for at least the last decade (if ever), a decade in which community care policies have been discussed and encouraged as the conventional wisdom, following the publication of the White Paper 'Better services for the Mentally Ill'[1] in 1975, which was itself predated by the 1959 Mental Health Act. Sir Henry Yellowlees discusses the obstacles to implementation in greater detail in his contribution to this volume.

Political issues

The crushing Conservative victory of June 1987 gave the Tory Government a large majority to ensure passage of its legislative program and continuation of its policy of reducing public expenditure.

Violence seems to be on the increase, both in domestic and social settings, with escalating child-abuse, wife battering, and divorce rates, as well as increases in drug, solvent and alcohol abuse. Street violence and riot have happened in several British cities, the equivalent of 'Watts' in the United States the 1960s. All this has been the staple fare of informed and journalistic comment for at least a decade. Overcrowding in the prisons is now so great that 'roof-top protests' are almost routine happenings.

Quality of the public services

Confidence in the State education sector plummeted after a prolonged bitter strike, and the daily diet of newspaper stories about the failings of personal social service departments and local authority housing departments to cope with their respective problems, presents a picture of the State in general and the Welfare State in particular, being under siege, if not in actual decay. Concern about conditions in long-stay hospitals, (generated in the 1960s with the exposure of bad practices) has been replaced by anxiety about the plight of the mentally ill in bed-and-breakfast accommodation without proper day care.

The decline in Britain's manufacturing output has given rise to serious concern and, in 1983, for the first time ever, there was a trade deficit on manufactured goods which mushroomed in 1988/9.[2] If one adds to this the problem of long-term unemployment (which remains high despite recent reduction) and the high cost of the social security budget, which also has to cope with the rise in the numbers of the 'old' old, 'crisis' seems too mild a descriptor.

Challenges to the Welfare State

It seems that the political climate in which the social services have to operate is more hostile than at any time since 1948.[3] The Keynesian–Beveridge tradition has been criticized from two directions. The 'new right' ideology of individualism claims that the public provision of welfare services is wasteful and inefficient, and has failed to eradicate poverty and ill health and to reduce inequalities. On the other hand, the neo-Marxists argue that concepts of 'welfare' and 'capitalism' are incompatible and produce conflict, dramatically illustrated by the 'fiscal crisis'. The concept of Welfare is defended by the pragmatic, empirical but idealist policy makers and administrators. The 'new right' see this defence as professional self-interest and a burden on the economy. The neo-marxists are critical of any perspective or political action which appears to ignore the materialist facts.

Challenges to professional practice

A simultaneous, but unconnected, two-pronged attack on professionalism has further undermined confidence in the public social services. This attack has come from a government whose policy of attacking monopolies has resulted in breaking that of the opticians to dispense, with the result that there is 'High Street' commercial trading in spectacles, unknown in the United Kingdom since 1948. Solicitors no longer have a monopoly in conveyancing property, and the right of general medical practitioners to prescribe any drug has been curtailed or 'limited'. This attack by Government on professional expertise has been complicated by a

considerable disillusionment with professional performance on the part of the
informed general public as well as by the traditional conflict between bureaucratic
efficiency and professional independence. The deprofessionalizers (Illich, 1975;
Kennedy, 1981) those who question the basic assumptions behind medical practice,
support an increase in self-care and co-operatives. They have also stimulated a
growing and profound distrust of the language, techniques and outcomes of
professional intervention.

Allied to consumerism, and a half-understood and undigested notion of
professional activity as mystification of the everyday world, the last decade,
certainly in the United Kingdom, has been an uncomfortable one for that
traditional world of professional activity in which debates have customarily taken
place about changes in techniques, delivery systems and professional values within
the profession itself, and away from outside intervention. Even the conservative
United Kingdom Law Society has had to respond to public criticism of its
regulatory techniques.

Society in crisis?

This schematic outline suggests a society in profound crisis, with no common
values, and conflict rather than consensus and compromise in public affairs. It
implies the surprising absence of a common culture (in a society with a relatively
small population, contained on an island, with diminishing overseas responsibilities
and with a common language). The NHS in general, and mental health care in
particular, have to be seen against this background.

Yet there is a civic or public culture about which there is consensus. Forty years
after the original debate about the role of the State in a universal commitment to
publicly provided services, all the survey data show strong support for this kind
of commitment and provision and the NHS consistently comes out with the
highest level of support (Harrison & Gretton, 1985).[7] Even the NHS, however, is
now under considerable threat from the Government 1989 White Paper.

Public expenditure

With a faltering, if not declining, economy,[4] public expenditure trends have
become a consistent and disputed area of political debate. One authoritative review
(Gillion & Hemming, 1985) had described the United Kingdom economy thus:

> The period between 1975 and 1981 saw a slow down in both economic growth
> (real Gross Domestic Product) and the growth of social expenditure (in cost
> terms) in all countries, with the United Kingdom growth rate in both cases
> remaining the lowest.

This continues ...

> However the UK is the only country in which the health share of social spending
> has not increased over this period.

The official Government statement has this to say ...

> The cash plans mean that public spending between 1985–86 and 1988–89 should
> be held broadly stable in real terms. It is expected to fall in relation to the nation's
> income and by 1988–89 to be the lowest proportion since 1972–73, with or
> without privatisation proceeds.[5]

It is also clear that there is a consistent decline in total government expenditure as
a percentage of GDP; since 1982–83 the assumption made by government is that
the economy will continue to grow slowly, but with the percentage used for public
expenditure falling from $44\frac{1}{2}$% in 1985–86 (the lowest since 1979–80) to 41%
in 1988–89 (the lowest since 1972–73.)[6]

Health expenditure

Total health care expenditure in the United Kingdom as a percentage of GDP has
risen slowly since the inception of the NHS, and, in almost every year since the
mid-1950s, faster than the rest of the economy.[7] The Office of Health Economics
correctly interprets these figures as suggesting that the United Kingdom
spends proportionately 25% less annually of its wealth on health than other
comparable countries over the late 1970s and early 1980s. Thus there has been a
significant change since 1960 when the United Kingdom was one of the largest
spenders in the OECD.

If we turn to the gross costs of the NHS in the United Kingdom we see a rise
in current spending from £8,732 billion in 1979–80 to £16,467 billion in 1985–86
and a rise in capital expenditure over the same period from £496 million to £962
million.[8] Another way of looking at health expenditure is to compare the figures
for the first year of NHS operation (1949) with those of the early 1980s. Taking
the 1949 gross cost of £437m as 100, by 1984 the figure had risen (in terms of
1949 prices) to £1581m, or 320, so that the cost has trebled. In the same period,
the NHS increased its share of GNP from 3·9% in 1949 to 6·2% in 1984.[9] At the
same time health has had to compete with other publicly provided services
(housing, education and especially social security and unemployment benefits) and
the percentage of United Kingdom public expenditure going to health increased
by one-seventh; that to defence declined by about one third; to housing, declined
by one-third; to education, increased by one-third; and to social security, increased
by 100%.[10]

The major share, about 60% of this expenditure, has continued to go to the
hospital services over this period, with the other parts of the Service, family
practitioners, pharmaceuticals, opticians, dental care and community-based services
sharing the balance. About 6% of health expenditure goes on hospital and
community services for the mentally ill (in-, out- and day-patient care) and about
1% of the personal social services budget is used for residential and day-care
services.[11] Since the NHS is a major employer (of about one million people) the

gross cost of salaries and wages (excluding family doctors, opticians and dentists) accounted for 45% in 1954, 51% in 1974 and 52% in 1984 of total expenditure. It also owns 50,000 acres of land, 2,000 hospitals of various sizes, health centres, clinics, laundries, ambulance stations and residential homes, with an estimated capital replacement cost of £21,000m at 1983 prices.[12]

The sources of finance for the service have remained virtually unchanged over the years, despite the current government's flirtation with insurance. In 1985–86, 82% of NHS finance came from taxation, compared with 11% from national insurance contributions and 3% from charges. The sheer volume of support from general taxation shows how impervious the service is to alternative forms of finance.[13]

The political context of administrative developments

Despite 13 changes of government from 1946 to 1990 there has been general agreement about the aims of the Service throughout this period. These were restated in general terms by the Royal Commission[14] and subsequently by the government in its public expenditure plans for 1986. For our purposes the most significant point in the latter is the fifth one; to

> continue to improve community support by strengthening primary care and community health and social services for people who do not require continuing hospital care.[15]

This is clearly relevant to improvement in these services. As Maynard & Bosanquet (1986) point out, 'managers in the NHS face a problem of how to turn these policy objectives into specific and costed programmes.' It is this problem that links the economic with the political and administrative history of the NHS in general and the fate of the mental health services in particular.

Fifty years ago Lord Horder, in a foreword to the famous PEP Report 'Britain's Health', (Mervyn Herbert, 1939), wrote that 'Health is hammering at the door of economics'. General acceptance of public financing of health services was the result of the serious underfinancing of the earlier voluntary system, revealed during the War. More recently (1983) Theodore Marmor has reminded us that 'medical care finance is dominated by public expenditure' and he puts it even more succinctly in his Proposition 5 in his contribution to this volume.[16] Horder's warning and Marmor's axiom are separated by what might be called Beveridge's promise and Eckstein's foresight.

Beveridge gave a hostage to fortune in two short paragraphs.[17] The first was that there should be 'a national health service for the prevention and cure of disease and disability by medical treatment.' The second should send a shiver down the spine of any health service manager. It is an open-ended, uncosted, value-laden statement; that there should be

> a comprehensive national health service which will ensure that for every citizen

there is available whatever medical treatment he requires, in whatever form he requires it, domiciliary or institutional, general, specialist or consultant, and will ensure also the provision of dental, ophthalmic and surgical appliances, nursing and midwifery and rehabilitation after accidents. Whether or not payment towards the cost of the health service is included in the social insurance contribution, the service itself should:

(i) be organised not by the Ministry concerned with social insurance but by the Department responsible for the health of the people and for positive and preventive as well as curative measures.

(ii) be provided where needed without contribution conditions in any individual case.

The early problems of the NHS

Thus Beveridge was responsible for making the deliberate distinction between those government departments responsible for social security payments and health care delivery, and for the destruction of the relationship between health needs and the ability to pay for medical care, and despite the opposition to the proposals in the White Paper and the Parliamentary Bill from the British Medical Association (BMA), these two principles were incorporated into legislation.[18] Beveridge's biographer, Jose Harris (1977), describes how euphorically the Report was received by the general public, but she also reminds us that it was more than just a recommendation about a free NHS; it was also about a system of family allowances, social insurance and a government commitment to full employment.

Much of the hidden agenda and implicit assumptions about the health service in the United Kingdom rest upon whether or not Beveridge's promises could have been or should be fulfilled. Within ten years of the inception of the Service, Eckstein was able to claim, with some justification, that

> the health services were now wed, for better or worse, to the national budgetary process and that it had become almost overnight, and would continue to be, the chief claimant on civil expenditure and along with this, the first target of any objective or emotionally felt need for economy on a national scale (Eckstein, 1958).

The NHS inherited a dilapidated and disorganised array of medical services, along with staff loyalties to the pre-war way of administering the service, which was to produce 'vexatious political pressures and frustrating personal relationships within the service' (Eckstein, 1958). In his contribution to this volume, Yellowlees gives examples of the continuation of these pressures and relationships in the Health Service of the 1980s. There was discontent within the NHS between 1948 and the 1960s, mainly on the part of GPs who were dissatisfied with their remuneration, the nature of their contracts and the state of their practice premises. The major political issues were, however, conflicts surrounding the imposition of prescription charges in 1951, with Bevan and Wilson resigning from the

Government on this, and the inquiry into the cost of the Service in 1956[19] (Guillebaud) which reported that the service was under financial control, giving value for money and treating more patients. It nevertheless warned against rising expectations, the changing demographic structure and the consequent demands on the service and, in a little-read minority note, raised the question of the lack of integration between the parts of the service.

Administrative panacea

However, once the Ministry of Health and the Ministry of Pensions and National Insurance were merged into the new Department of Health and Social Security (DHSS), 1966, a 'super' ministry, government attention turned to the original tripartite administrative structure, the legacy of Bevan's compromise. This gave added impetus to the idea of integrating the three parts of the service. Attempts at reorganisation in 1968 and 1970 fell under medical opposition and it was left to a Conservative Government to construct an integrated Health Service. This was heavily criticized as being too bureaucratic, inflexible, hierarchical and prone to duplicate planning and delivery of services at various levels. This was only one of the many criticisms the Service was facing, and the Royal Commission which was set up to find answers did not hesitate to recommend the abolition of the middle tier (the Area Health Authority). This was carried out in 1982.

Authority and power

The organizational structure of the NHS, and thus the distribution of 'authority' within the organization, is decided by the statutory power of the Secretary of State after consultation with professional and other interest groups. The Secretary of State also controls the second resource, 'money', laying down the principles of distribution, such as the formula put forward by the Resource Allocation Working Party (RAWP). This will be explained in more detail later. His authority and the large-scale decisions he appears to be taking cannot necessarily be made effective. District Health Authority (DHA) members, although appointed by the Secretary of State through the Region, are not obliged to follow his instructions unless he issues a directive in writing, except in terms of keeping within their budget.

Central/local relations

There is conflict between the centre and the locality, a conflict that has always been a part of nearly every aspect of British political and social life. The Department of Health (formerly DHSS) and the Regional Health Authorities often seem to be in opposition to local priorities which the district HAs may claim are legitimate. The processes of Annual Review, efficiency measures, privatization, the continued existence of RAWP and the struggle for 'developments' add to this pressure and conflict between central and local authorities. At the local level, with funding restricted by cash limits, competition between the acute and the 'Cinderella' services is inevitable. Centrally generated priorities and policies do not necessarily become translated into local services through the collaboration of DHAs and local authorities. Again Yellowlees' paper gives clear examples of the difficulties of planning between local authorities and health authorities.[20]

There is often hostility between health authorities and local authority social service departments over joint funding, which is the constitutional requirement to co-operate, collaborate and develop services for the same client groups. These arrangements are insufficient to overcome the suspicion between the two kinds of authority. This may be due in part to the different ways in which they are constituted, the health authorities (Regional and District) being nominated and the local councils being elected, as well as the difference in funding, with the former entirely dependent on central government finance, while the latter have a measure of autonomy with the power to raise local revenue through the rates. This power has been curtailed recently by central government, using the device of 'rate capping', that is to say, restricting the amount of money that can be raised in this way. This has led to legal disputes where the 'capping' has been challenged in the courts. In a resource-constrained environment, both groups of public agencies find it difficult to entrust their clients to an alternative administration over which they have no control and to which they have to donate some of their own scarce resources. Marmor elegantly describes this process in the following way:[21]

> Where fragmentation is structural and continuing, the obvious incentive is different. It is to 'externalise' the costs to other jurisdictions and to 'internalise' administrative responsibility.

Responsibility

The reorganization of 1974 tried to make a definite distinction between medical and nonmedical areas of work, and problems arise because there are bound to be overlaps and difficulties in making this distinction in the care of the mentally handicapped, the elderly and the mentally ill. Disagreements about caring strategies and low ideological consensus give rise to negative views by agencies of each other's work and worth. Collaboration can work if there is consensus or agreed demarcation rules about the forms of care for priority groups. Social workers in both general- and psychiatric hospitals are funded by local (nonhealth) authorities although they are dealing with health service clients. Thus working relationships and lines of communication between professional health workers and semiprofessional social workers can be difficult. Clear examples of this are described in Yellowlees' paper.

The importance of geography

There is no automatic geographical coterminosity between authorities. Although the 1974–82 Area HA boundaries were intended to match with boroughs and counties, this principle disappeared when the AHA's were abolished in 1982. The four Regional Health Authorities for London are good examples of this mismatch, with considerable cross-boundary patient flows but no financial compensation.

Centrally determined priorities

The two most recent reviews of Conservative and Labour government policy since 1970 conclude

1. that 'policy towards health and social security over this period exhibited much greater continuity than is commonly supposed (Atkinson, Hills & Legrand, 1986),' and
2. that 'the course of events has been complex: it has not resulted from a simple policy imperative, as much of the popular political debate suggests' (Robinson, 1986).

Both Labour and Conservative Governments of the 1970s and 1980s have committed themselves to the redistribution of resources, the ordering of priorities and cost containment policies within the service. All three have proved difficult to implement in spite of widespread acceptance of the principles behind them.

First, changes in medical technology and therapeutic techniques have proved to be expensive and have dramatically raised public expectations in the last ten years.

Secondly, there has been an increasing strain on the traditional division between acute episodic medicine and chronic continuing care due to the increasing problem of the elderly in the population who are highly dependent on the service. The latest figures produced by the DHSS show a dramatic rise in the numbers being treated in geriatric hospitals (DHSS, 1976).

Thirdly, pressure groups and a number of well-publicized cases have drawn attention to the so-called Cinderella services, and there is now general agreement that the balance of resources should be adjusted in their favour.

Fourthly, there is a growing public as well as professional recognition that there are other inequalities in the operation of the NHS, involving differences of access, use and outcome between different social classes, debates about equality of opportunity for ethnic groups using the service, and gender differences in treatment and inequalities between different geographical areas.

These imbalances were the result of the policy of allocating resources mainly on the basis of existing provision when new facilities were commissioned (the Crossman formula, a single relationship between population and hospital beds dating from 1971). The 1976 RAWP formula was an attempt to redress these geographical imbalances. This formula resulted in 'over-provided' health authorities having their current and capital revenues restricted to a 'target', with those above target 'losing' revenue, and those below, gaining. In general, this meant that the North of England benefited at the expense of the South, with London being particularly hard hit. This is not the place to go into the details or the criticisms of RAWP.[22] The main losers were the London Teaching hospitals, who faced a gap between the population for whom they were required to plan and that which demanded the use of their services.

Richard Rose (1982) argued that social scientists and politicians find it difficult to agree about criteria for the distribution of public resources. He suggests four possible criteria, territorial, fiscal exchange, population and need. These are all unsatisfactory in their own way. Territorial distribution is rarely used because of the imbalance of population in the United Kingdom. Distribution by past fiscal contribution is an inegalitarian mode, simply giving to those who are already well endowed. Distribution according to population size might be acceptable if population were spread evenly throughout the country. Distribution according to need moves policy makers from technical to normative and political criteria. ·Government attempts to adhere to the RAWP formula illustrate the difficulty of choosing between these criteria.

The publication of RAWP coincided with a more general recognition of the problems of chronic and mental illness and a consequent decline in the power of the consultants in the more glamorous specialties so that the 'cinderella services' began to take a larger share of NHS resources from 1976. The 1979 Conservative Government continued with RAWP and appeared quite unafraid to take on the London teaching hospitals. This same Government adhered to the priorities as stated in the 1976 Document (DHSS, 1976) that is, that there should be a redistribution in the direction of the elderly, the mentally handicapped and the mentally ill. The Government also continued, albeit with adaptations, the planning system of 1976, and thereafter allocated resources according to Operational and Strategic plans, later replaced by annual planning reviews, which have to be in line with 'prevailing national policies and priorities, as well as areas of local priority (DHSS, 1982).

The planning system thus allows, in theory, the central administration to control the local one, enforces priorities and allows cost containment policies to dominate strategic thinking. In this, the present Government simply took over the cash limit system from the 1974–79 Labour Administration. This allocates revenue on a yearly basis to all 192 district health authorities via the 14 Regional HAs for England and Wales, and reduces the revenue accordingly if there has been an overspend. The introduction, in 1983, of the Griffiths' idea of general managers was intended to provide one point of authority within a district (the District General Manager), or region (the Region General Manager), from which all decisions on a day-to-day basis will emanate (Carrier & Kendall, 1986).

The DHSS had a similar managerial approach at the top with the Health Services Supervisory Board and the NHSS Management Board. The General Manager and the Unit General Managers in charge of the district carry out policy decided by district members. These members are appointed by the Region and the Minister, usually in the following proportions; four from the local authority, usually with clear party political allegiance, two from the relevant University, a Consultant to represent consultant staff, a GP, a nurse and a trade union member, and six generalist members. However, it is clear from the DHSS Circular HC (81) 6 (Appendix 1 para. g) that

> No member is appointed to represent a sectional or personal interest. It is important that members contribute in a constructive as well as a questioning way to the whole work of the authority, avoiding the temptation to concentrate on matters of a particular personal interest. ... Members must, therefore, be prepared to recognise not only the duty of the Authority to reach decisions, but also the corporate responsibility of the members for those decisions once taken.

Decision-making in the NHS is, however, far removed from this simple admonition and can dramatically affect the approval and implementation of priorities, especially where more than one agency is involved in care of a client group.

The political and economic climate for community care

The present Government has introduced a number of measures which produce conflict in local health services and put strain on policies for the care of mentally ill people. By placing pressure on local services at the same time as redistributing resources to new priority groups hostility is deflected on to the very services that require support, changing attitudes and concrete resources. The fiat on efficiency savings, manpower controls and short-term programmes makes it difficult to take action to improve priority services.

Efficiency savings are exhibited as cash reduction to allocation which places managers in the position of reducing resources while attempting to maintain services. 'Man-power reductions' in 1983 attempted to slim down the professional, semiprofessional and ancillary labour forces. Short-term programmes are intended to be a form of self-financing, using projected efficiency savings for necessary developments. Finally, the DHSS insisted that the Districts put their hotel services (laundry, catering and domestic) out to competitive tender, raising the spectre of industrial relations conflicts as public service labour unions resist redundancies and job losses. Thus the political and economic climate is far from ideal for developing a positive program of community care, in spite of clear statements of priority from successive governments and their commitment to a comprehensive range of psychiatric services at a local level. Successive Ministers of Health[23] have placed mental health high on the agenda. Statements of government intentions have emphasised the need for consultation, collaboration and co-operation between the voluntary and statutory services outside the NHS, that is, the personal social services, employment and housing.

As we have seen the reorganization of local government and the NHS in 1974 transferred all aspects of health service management to health authorities while the non-health service functions were given to county and borough councils. The need for co-operation between the NHS and local government was clearly recognized in all the consultation papers leading up to reorganization. Joint consultative committees (JCCs) were set up to facilitate co-operation and the flow of money between authorities. Since 1976–77 about £623 million has been allocated to joint finance, and health authorities have been allowed to transfer joint finance resources freely between capital and revenue.[24]

The 1980 Care in the Community programme stressed the importance of joint finance so that programmes could be jointly agreed upon between health and social service departments but financial constraints (Cash limits, etc) made this flow difficult to implement, and raise areas of conflict between central and local authorities, and between health authorities and local authorities.

Mental health policy in the UK

The 'Better Services for the Mentally Ill' White Paper (1975)[25], the Nodder Report (1978) and 'Care in Action' Consultation Document (DHSS, 1981) form the basis of mental health policy in the United Kingdom.

'Better Services' laid down norms of provision, attempting to match resources to needs. Nodder argued for the creation of Psychiatric Management Teams, to bring some unity into the health and social services setting by making a team responsible for monitoring standards and quality of care. 'Care in Action' identified four main tasks as follows.

1. The building up of local psychiatric services in districts where provision was limited.

2. A commitment that every district should have suitable provision for the increasing numbers of elderly people with psychiatric disorders, ensuring that each district would have a consultant psychiatrist with a special interest in elderly people.

3. To make satisfactory arrangements for the closure of badly placed mental hospitals.

4. For the local authority social service departments, with voluntary bodies and health authorities to provide the necessary residential and day-care facilities and other support and rehabilitation services.

By 1981 there was growing evidence that these tasks were not being successfully undertaken in many areas. The shift of the balance of care from the NHS to local authorities and of resources to priority groups was happening far more slowly than had been hoped. These objectives were reiterated in the 1984 DHSS Annual Report. Following this, the 1983 Mental Health Act emphasized the civil liberties of detained patients and the importance of social work in this area.

The Second Report of the Social Services Committee; Community Care, 1985–86[26] was concerned with the question of whether Community Care has become a reality.

> We do not wish to slow down the exodus from mental illness or mental handicap hospitals for its own sake, but we do look to see the same degree of Ministerial pressure, and the provision of the necessary resources, devoted to the creation of alternative services. Any fool can close a long stay hospital; it takes more time and trouble to do it compassionately. [para 40]

The committee went on to say

> the Minister must ensure that mental illness or mental handicap hospital provision is not reduced without demonstrably adequate alternative services being provided beforehand for those discharged from hospital and for those who would otherwise seek admission.

This suggests that a range of practices and policies are possible. It is difficult to define what is 'demonstrably adequate'. Norms, good practices and availability of resources are involved. The concept of alternative services is also open to discussion and there is no general acceptance among medical and social service professionals about the implications of such a statement. 'Care in Action', 'Care in the Community', joint finance, funding and consultation all suggest that resources will be going (with the patients) from the health services to the social service departments in the form of dowries (running costs) or that there will be joint finance from central government. This in turn implies that most patients will never need to return to hospital, that hostels are no worse than hospitals for the purpose of decent living conditions and that social service departments will be able to cope with the effects of rate capping.

In 1985 the Government published its response to the House of Commons Community Care Report. It contained the following important statement

> The Government confirms its commitment to the development of the integrated network of central policies and local services necessary for community care, and its priority for mentally ill and mentally handicapped people. It will continue to allocate resources with that development and that priority in mind, and to impress on statutory authorities their responsibilities for joint planning and joint use of resources to achieve the same priority developments. It will use its influence on service and management structures and central arrangements for audit, inspection, monitoring and evaluation (including the Health Advisory Service, the National Development Team for Mentally Handicapped People and the Social Services Inspectorate to disseminate and encourage good practice.)

Conclusion

There has been a decline in the numbers of patients in long-stay mental hospitals. The quality of alternative services and the speed with which they can be provided to match the decline in inpatient numbers are the two dominant concerns. The main difficulty in providing high-quality services in sufficient quantity has been:

1. lack of economic growth in Britain and the public expenditure cutbacks.
2. the difficulty of redistributing health service resources away from the historically dominant areas of the service towards designated priorities.
3. the complexity of the collaborative machinery involving co-operation between different professional and semiprofessional groups, and different administrative and funding agencies.
4. the negotiable quality of local decision-making and the uncertainty of its outcome.

These obstacles are or have been a constant feature within the NHS and other caring agencies and their presence will continue to act as a brake on the community care of mentally ill people.

The NHS in general, and mental health policies and services in particular, are operating in a political and economic context which is unhelpful and obstructive. The 'cold economic climate' (Abel Smith, 1981) of the last six years has led to competition for resources between independently legitimate services.

Health care policy in the United Kingdom since the Second World War shows a large measure of consistency. Policies for health care need to be politically acceptable, economically feasible and administratively viable. The first may have been so for some time but so far the second and third have not proved to be so simple. Under the Labour Governments of 1948, 1966 and 1976 the main thrust of health care policy was directed towards *rationalizing* the administration of the service, *reorganizing* the central departments into one ministry (the DHSS), and *redistributing* resources (RAWP). Every health minister, since Iain Macleod in the 1950s, has considered mental health policy to be important but it is only since 1976 that it has become an official priority.

Under Conservative Governments, the process can be described as one of *centralizing* decision-making (1974 reorganization), *controlling* resources (strict cash limits and man-power controls from 1982 onwards) and *containing* costs through efficiency savings and self-funding.

The 1981 'Care in Action' and 'Care in the Community' Documents emphasized the collaborative arrangements which should operate between health and personal social service departments, and had been in existence since 1973. Although critics may be sceptical about the reality of community care, at least mental health is established on the medicopolitical agenda. The greater emphasis given to mental health policy is due to the realization that earlier forms of care are no longer appropriate because of developments in drug therapy and a better understanding of the nature of mental illness. There is also greater awareness of the size and scale of the population affected by the presence and quality of mental health services, heightened by a number of scandals in long-stay institutions (Martin, 1984) and the attempt of professionals, semiprofessionals and laymen to socialize somatic conditions thus drawing attention to the inappropriateness of hospitals for care. Hospitals as 'asylums' have had the advantage of visibility, 'solidity', presence and professional justification for their existence. The concept of 'Community' is a more nebulous, invisible, abstract phenomenon, high on values but low on operational definition. Local administrators, as well as health and local authority members, have considerable room to negotiate methods of delivering services, within the parameters of limited resources.

Both the political and economic contexts of mental health care are unstable, uncertain and unpredictable. Social divisions have deepened in the past few years, fuelled by unemployment and disappointed aspirations. The assumptions underpinning the National Health Service are also under political and economic scrutiny. It is '*National*' because it is centrally funded and legitimized, but in practice, it is locally administered and still subject to immense variation in standards, commitments and resources; '*Health*' yet it concentrates mainly on the cure of disease rather than the promotion of health; and still a '*Service*' despite the fact that it is becoming increasingly subject to market principles, with the introduction of efficiency drives and measurable performance objectives and indicators. If the future looks bleak for the NHS in general, how much bleaker must it look for community care which depends on those same principles. Despite all this there has been consensus, about aims and priorities in general, over the past 40 years; although they have been difficult to put into practice, they have been given constant reinforcement from the centre. The wide support for the NHS and the concept of community care means that publicly provided services of this kind are likely to remain in the centre of political debate.

Postscript
The Audit Commission and the Griffiths Review
The Audit Commission published a report (DHSS, 1986) on a variety of community care schemes. This concluded that all the successful schemes involved 'a radical departure from the generally accepted ways of doing things'. In particular, they showed six features.

1. The presence of strong and committed local 'champions' of change.
2. A focus on action not bureaucratic machinery.
3. Locally integrated machinery for service planning purposes.
4. A focus on the local neighbourhood.

5.   A multiprofessional team approach.

6.   A partnership between statutory services and voluntary organizations.

The obstacles to implementation adduced by Sir Henry Yellowlees (Chap. 12, this volume) are all borne out in this Review by the Audit Commission, and the absence of these obstacles is indicative of successful community care schemes.

At the same time the Government announced the appointment of Sir Roy Griffiths, Mrs Thatcher's health service adviser, to undertake a review of community care. This was a response, not to the good practices highlighted by the Audit Commission, but to its criticism that the care of the mentally ill, the mentally handicapped and the elderly suffered through the waste of resources, estimated at £6 billion. As mentioned, the Griffiths' Report recommended that the responsibility for community care should lie with local authorities, and this may be why the Report was virtually ignored by the government which commissioned it until a statement by the Secretary of State in July 1989.

During the 1987 General Election campaign there was hardly a single mention of mental health care. Almost all the attention given to the NHS concentrated on the length of the waiting lists for acute and non-acute surgery; the role of the private sector in competing with or complementing the NHS, and an acrimonious dispute about the level of spending by the Conservative Government since 1979. None of the Manifestoes estimated the costs of community care. Mrs Thatcher's Conservative party won a landslide victory, for a third term of office. The July 1989 statement referred to above promised a White Paper on Community Care, to be implemented in 1991. But community care policies are endangered by implications of the 1989 White Paper on the NHS which appear incompatible with recommendations of the Griffiths Report.

Notes

1. Department of Health and Social Security (1975). *Better Services for the Mentally Ill*, White Paper. Cmnd 6233. HMSO.
2. House of Lords (1975). *Report of the Select Committee on Overseas Trade*. HMSO. *See also* Lord Aldington (1986). Britain's Manufacturing Industry. *Royal Bank of Scotland Review*, **151** September.
3. A similar point is made in an Irish Government Report. (1986). *Report of the Commission on Social Welfare*. Dublin Stationery Office.
4. Central Statistical Office (March–September 1986) *Economic Trends. 389–96* HMSO. (In **389** p. 37, in March 1986, Seasonally adjusted unemployment was over 3 million with under 200,000 vacancies.)
5. *The Government's Expenditure Plans* (1986). Vol I *Cmnd 9702*. HMSO.
6. As Note 5.
7. OECD (1985). *Measuring Health Care 1960–1983*. OECD Paris. Quoted in OHE (1986). *Health Expenditure in the UK*. Office of Health Economics.
8. As Note 5.

9. As Note 7.
10. As Note 7.
11. House of Commons (1986). *Fourth Report from the Social services Committee 1985–6 Public Expenditure on the Social Services*, Vol I HMSO.
12. DHSS (1983). *Health Care and its Costs* HMSO.
13. As Cmnd 9702 (Note 5) p. 212.
14. DHSS (1979). *Report of the Royal Commission on the NHS Cmnd 9615*. HMSO.
15. As Note 5.
16. Marmor, T. (1983). *Political Analysis and American Medical Care*. Cambridge University Press.
17. Beveridge, Sir W. (1942). *Social Insurance and Allied Services*. (Paras 426–7) *Cmnd 6404*, HMSO.
18. Foot, M. (1975). *Aneurin Bevan*. Paladin. Willcocks, A. J. (1967). *The Creation of the NHS*. Routledge and Kegan Paul. Klein, R. (1983). *The Politics of the NHS*. Longman. Pater, J. (1981). *The Making of the NHS*. King Edward's Hospital Fund for London.
19. Guillebaud, C. (1956). *Report of a Committee of Inquiry into the Cost of the NHS, Cmnd 9663*. HMSO.
20. Yellowlees, Sir H., his contribution to this Volume pp. 167–178.
21. See p. 137–153 Marmor's contribution to this Volume.
22. DHSS (1976). *Report of the Resource Allocation Working Party (RAWP) Sharing Resources for Health in England*. HMSO. *See also* Carrier, J. (1978). Positive Discrimination in the Allocation of NHS Resources. In (Brown, M. & Baldwin, S. ed.) *The Year Book of Social Policy in Britain 1985–6*. Routledge and Kegan Paul.
23. There were nine Ministers of Health from 1951–1956, and six Secretaries of State for Social Services since then. Ian Macleod, Derek Walker Smith and Enoch Powell, Conservatives, & Richard Crossman and David Ennals, Labour have shown the most interest in Mental Health Policy.
24. *Fourth Report* as Note 11.
25. *Better Services* as Note 1.
26. DHSS (1985). *Government Response to the Second Report from the Social Services Committee 1984–85 Session. Community Care, with special reference to adult mentally ill and mentally handicapped people. Cmnd 9674*. HMSO.

References

Abel Smith, B. (1981). Health Care in a Cold Economic Climate. *The Lancet*, 14 Feb.

Atkinson, A. B., Hills, J. & Legrand, J. (1986). *The Welfare State in Britain, 1970–1985; Extent and Effectiveness*. STICERD: London.

Carrier, J. & Kendall, I. (1986). NHS Management and the Griffiths Report. In (Brenton, M. & Ungerson, C. ed.).*The Year Book of Social Policy In Britain 1985–6*. Routledge: Kegan Paul.

DHSS (1976). *Priorities for Health and Social Services in England. A Consultative Document*. HMSO.

DHSS (1981). *Consultative Document: Care in Action* HMSO.

DHSS (1981). *Health Services Management: the Membership of District Health Authorities HC (81) 6* (Appendix 1 para g) HMSO.

DHSS (1982). *Health Services Development; the NHS Planning System.* Health Circular HC (82) 6.

DHSS Nodder, T. (1978). *Organisational and Management Problems of Mental Illness Hospitals.* HMSO.

DHSS (1986). *Making a Reality of Community Care. A Report by the Audit Commission.* HMSO.

Eckstein, H. (1958). *The English Health Service.* Harvard University Press, Cambridge, Mass.

Gillion, C. & Hemming, R. (1985). Social Expenditure in the United Kingdom in a Comparative Context; Trends, Explanations and Projections. In (Klein, R. & O'Higgins, M. ed.). *The Future of Welfare.* Blackwell: Oxford.

The Government Statistical Service (1987). *NHS Hospital Acute In-patient Statistics – England 1974–85.* DHSS.

Hall, P., Land, H., Parker, R. & Webb, A. (1975). *Change Choice and Conflict in Social Policy.* Heineman Educational Books.

Harris, J. (1977). *William Beveridge, a Biography.* Oxford University Press.

Harrison, A. & Gretton, J. (1985). *Health Care UK; an Economic Social and Policy Audit* pp. 35–46. Chartered Institute of Public Finance and Accountancy.

Herbert, Mervyn, S. (1939). *Britain's Health.* Penguin Books.

Holmes, M. (1986). *The First Thatcher Government.* Harvester Press.

House of Commons (1985). *The Second Report of the Social Services Committee, Community Care.* HMSO.

Illich, I. (1975). *Medical Nemesis The Expropriation of Health.* Marion Boyars.

Kennedy, I. (1981). *The Unmasking of Medicine.* Allen and Unwin.

Maynard, A. & Bosanquet, B. (1986). *Public Expenditure on the NHS: Recent Trends and Future Problems.* Institute of Health Service Managers & British Medical Association.

Martin, J. P. (1984). *Hospitals in Trouble.* Blackwell: Oxford.

Robinson, R. (1986). Restructuring the Welfare State; in Analysis of Public Expenditure, 1979/80–1984/4. *The Journal of Social Policy,* **15** Part 1 (Jan).

Rose, R. (1982). *Understanding the United Kingdom.* Longman: London.

10

The political and economic context of mental health care in the United States

Theodore R. Marmor & Karyn Gill

The American mental health 'industry' has vastly changed since World War II. There has been dramatic growth in the use and costs of mental health services, the variety of these services, the places where they are provided, and the number and type of specialized mental health personnel. This chapter first briefly reviews the background to these changes and the trends in mental health care over the past 30 years. Its second part analyses the ways in which American politics – its structure and culture – shapes the formulation of 'problems', the options considered, and the forms of policy that can be realistically implemented. Its purpose is to illuminate how the cross-nationally familiar forms of mental illness and treatment are constrained by the American political system.

Analysis of trends

Recent trends in mental health service delivery in both the United States and the United Kingdom are well known. Historically sequestered at home or in jails and workhouses, a substantial proportion of the severely mentally ill have been transferred during this century from large public hospitals to care provided in community clinics, nursing homes, and general hospitals. The pressures for these changes, as noted particularly in the chapters by Katschnig and by Leff, have been numerous. The most prominent examples include the 'deinstitutionalization' strategies of the 1960s and the judicial interventions on behalf of the mentally ill, in particular those of the 1970s.

Since the mid-1970s, however, the overriding American concern in this area has been the impact on the mentally ill of the fiscal contractions of a budget-cutting era. In 1980, the United States spent 7.5% of total health care expenditures, or $20 billion, on mental health services.[1] Between 1977 and 1980, the share of GNP devoted to mental health expenses decreased by 28%.[2] This decline has continued into the 1980s and can be expected to continue. The largest proportion of the mental health dollar is now spent in institutions that care for the mentally ill, while the largest proportion of the patient population receives treatment in clearly underfunded outpatient settings. And the size of the mentally ill population continues to grow as the 'baby boom' generation matures. This mismatch between patient needs and the delivery and financing of services results in severe strain as policy players scramble for a smaller share of the national health care financial 'pie'.[3]

But why should this be so when the percentage of United States GNP devoted to health care generally continues to rise? Traditionally, mental disorders have been viewed as 'different' from physical disorders. The causes are mysterious, cures rare, and victims afflicted with social stigma. Frequently, the medical establishment treats the physical problems related to these diseases, while neglecting the less tangible underlying problems.

One of the major problems in constructing policy options for mental health care is the very nature of mental disease and the delivery system required for its treatment. Many private health insurance companies resist comprehensive coverage of mental illness. They hesitate because the 'subjective' definition of conditions requiring care, the duration of treatment, and the criteria for recovery all challenge traditional insurance conventions. They believe it is actuarially difficult to measure risks without a predictable course of illness and regard the costs of long-term treatments as too unpredictable to be borne by private insurance.[4]

The models used to deliver care to the mentally disordered reflect these difficulties.[5] For example, most acute psychiatric disorders are diagnosed and treated within a medical–psychiatric model, where team members work directly with a physician who is a psychiatrist. This is the pattern usually reimbursed by third-party health payment plans because costs can be defined (e.g. on an institutional *per diem* basis) and quality of care can be crudely certified through state or JCAH (Joint Commission on Accreditation of Health Care Organizations) certification procedures. Other models, which rely principally on psychologists, social workers, and educators using psychotherapy, behaviour therapy, or even social/educational interventions (e.g. in marital problems) treat very large numbers of the emotionally disturbed, but are often unable to receive direct reimbursement by traditional 'health' payment programs.[6]

As noted, the separation of 'health' and 'mental health' treatment systems has resulted in distinctive and often inappropriate patterns of care for the mentally ill. It is now realized that, as a result of deinstitutionalization, patients outside hospitals require many services that traditional mental health care providers are not equipped to give. The link to community support and social services programs is critical for the mentally ill patient if there is to be integration back into a society of work, education, and family/social relationships. Current patterns of American health finance do not support these links; this has contributed to the 'revolving door' syndrome, mental patients moving through the costly emergency rooms and psychiatric units of our nation's general hospitals.[7]

The trends in mental health services since the 1960s document the dramatic shift in locus of treatment from the state mental institutions to community care facilities. But, it is obvious that American funding practices for the mentally ill are not consistent with this mode of treatment. Community programs funded by Alcohol, Drug Abuse & Mental Health Administration (ADAMHA) were cut by 30% between 1980 and 1982, as Professor Klerman notes in his chapter (this volume). And, like private insurers, Medicare and Medicaid have distinctly institutional medical biases in their distribution of health care funds.

This poses especially acute dilemmas for severely mentally ill patients. First of all, prevaling trends suggest there will be more severely mentally ill people in the future.[8] If the institutional population is restricted and payment is severely limited for outpatient care, the level of socially disruptive behaviour will increase nationwide. Patients will continue to enter traditional medical institutions, such as general hospitals or nursing homes, where care is often expensive and inappropriate; or, many will be shunted into board and care homes, prisons, or onto the streets. This problem will be exacerbated if those with less severe disorders enter the formal mental health field for care or if the chronically mentally ill increase their utilization of existing services.[9]

Second, even when community services are available to the mentally ill, they are often targeted to those with nonpsychotic emotional disorders, and provided in large part by nonmedical professionals, who may or may not be skilled in the diagnosis and treatment of the chronic mentally ill. Services between the health and supportive social services sectors are often fragmented, so that comprehensive mental health care comparable to that provided within a single institution is unavailable. The less structured nature of this model further decreases the likelihood of third-party reimbursement.

Although most Americans with emotional problems do not utilize the formal mental health system, the number who do seek help from this sector has increased dramatically over the past 30 years. Mental health practice has shifted the most prominent site of care away from the state mental hospital to the community. The result is that a large majority of Americans receive mental health treatment as outpatients. Traditional health financing has not followed the patient to this outpatient location. The consequences are serious: skewed resource allocation and questionable care of the many severely mentally ill patients in the United States. The problems will worsen as traditional sources of health financing are strained, as the numbers of severely mentally ill in the general population increase, and as all categories of the mentally disabled seek more services provided by the formal mental health care sector.

The politics of mental health

The preceding portrait of American mental health contains few surprises. Its component elements have been discussed in other chapters of this volume. And the particular difficulties it highlights constitute some of the economic, administrative, and organizational barriers to the implementation of innovative approaches to American mental health care. Our concern here is to ask what the connections are between the trends identified and the larger context of American politics. In a world of familiar difficulties and internationally available technologies, what difference does it make that the context is American? What would the visitor from Mars need to know about American politics to make sense of the way problems are formulated in American mental health, options identified, and courses of action taken or rejected.

We will sketch some critical features of the American polity and propose five generalizations which affect any sector of public policy. Details of the particular world of mental health politics will be required to refine this necessarily broad brush portrait. But the general shape of American politics makes a large difference not only for what can be implemented but for what policy actions can even be seriously contemplated.

The most striking feature of American politics, viewed cross-nationally, is its pervasive fearfulness of concentrated authority. American are suspicious of government while holding moralistically high-minded standards for the conduct of public life. The American Constitution expresses this suspicion in its determined fragmentation of power and responsibility; it disperses the legitimate power to act both areally (federalism) and functionally (separation of powers). No visitor can fail to be struck with how diverse the coalition of actors are whose co-operation (or bargains) are required for concentrated action in American politics. For most of American history, the scope of government has been quite limited, the constraints of liberal politics taken for granted in deeply rooted fears of both socialism and traditional authoritarianism.[10]

In the late twentieth century America's ethos of limited, constrained government remains the accepted rhetoric. The nation has a very large civil service but a mixture of disdain for and suspicion of it. Only rarely is the American higher civil service respected as an elite corps – on the model of Britain, France, Sweden, or Japan. Yet the tasks of government – from huge pension and public health insurance programs to global defence and macroeconomic planning – are immensely difficult. Modern government calls for gifted planners and managers to negotiate program complexities and manage the processes of innovation – and American public life certainly has had distinguished examples. But our leading governmental institutions are without the benefits of great formal authority and respect. American society fragments into the complicated pressure groups and local constituencies of any modern nation. But the American polity remains rooted in a cast of mind appropriate to a commercial agrarian society, requiring the most minimal of governmental performance. It is not surprising, in this context, that the implementation of innovative programs in any area is difficult.[11]

There is a paradoxical feature of this combination of fragmentation, suspicion, government growth, and the rhetoric of constraint. The very fragmentation of the political jurisdictions invites innovative proposals. Many audiences rather than a tightly bound central authority increase the number of points where policy suggestion may be made. The dispersal of authority encourages proponents to separate finance from program administration, to suggest bargains where one unit of government pays and another administers, externalizing costs and internalizing benefits in the jargon of political economists. At the same time, the diffusion of effective authority markedly increases the opportunities to block action, to separate aspiration from effective remedy, to stimulate agreement on the 'problem' to be solved rather than the remedy to be implemented. In this sense, the structure of American politics rewards innovative proposals, but retards implementation.[12]

If American political structures are fragmented, British authority, by comparison, is unusually concentrated. The effect of a typical British national election is one party controlling both the executive and legislative authorities. Cabinet ministers are drawn from Parliament, they constitute members of a collective decision-making body, and can count, within broad limits, on speedy legislative enactment of proposals that command agreement within the party. In that sense, British national government is unified constitutionally and practically.

Equally important, that unity affects the incentives of all other actors within the political community. Since the capacity to decide is evident, the thrust of pressure group efforts is directed at what is decided, not whether to decide. That means implementation forecasts are rewarded, not reiterations of fundamental disagreement over whether or not to act in a given policy area. Attention is directed at governmental departments, not at Parliament; the question centres not on whether a policy matter is decidable, but whether the decisions taken are doable in practice. And for that reason, it is taken for granted that continuing, explicit dialogue with the other actors whose behaviour is affected by policy is called for.* This incorporation of pressure group considerations into policy deliberation is institutionalized most formally within Royal Commissions, where the question is what to do about an identified area, assuming that the government in power can act upon what they are persuaded to do. Whereas the role of commissions in America is as much to delay or to rouse the demand for action, the usual Royal

---

* This was not the case in the drawing up of the 1989 White Paper 'Working For Patients' (Editors)

Commissions of unified regimes function differently. They are part of the process of finding acceptable, implementable courses of action in which the ability to choose is not in question.[13]

Finally, it is worth noting that British politics include many cultural elements that augment rather than challenge authority. While parliamentary institutions evolved as checks on the arbitrary power of the Crown, the reach of parliamentary sovereignty is broad, extending into any area where consideration of community problems warrant the possibility of collective action. As shown in the chapter by Yellowlees, the range of mental illness and pressure groups in Britain is quite comparable to that in America; the character of the politics is quite different.

US politics hinders coordination

Proposition one: *The structure of American politics makes co-ordinated problem-solving by public authorities difficult both in principle and in practice.*

The fragmentation of decision-making is designed and structured so as to impede speedy and co-ordinated policy choice. It is no accident that the two houses of the national legislature – and of almost all the states – have varying electoral cycles and do their work under rules, party auspices, and committee arrangements that make co-ordination difficult. These features have their roots in constitutional principles and traditions that make the creation of an issue majority at any level of American politics extremely difficult. Such arrangements are directed against a powerful state; their rationale includes most prominently the fear of governmental coercion. In American politics a key tradeoff is between the capacity of the state to act quickly and with unity and the value of freedom from state authority: both separation of powers and complex federalism contribute to what might be called hobbled majoritarianism.

For most of American history, the fragmentation of American national government was largely irrelevant to mental health. The response to the mentally ill was clearly a state and local responsibility. The dispersion of authority that bore on mental health arose from the degree to which state and local authorities recreated the fragmentation of separated powers. In the post-World War II period, the complex interactions of both federalism and the competition of courts, legislatures, and executives shaped the governmental world dealing with mental health.[14]

Proposition two: *The deliberate fragmentation of American public authority conditions the treatment of all public policy issues.*

That fragmentation also produces at least three characteristic forms of political dispute – forms that reappear but with different distributions over time and within particular policy domains.

Issues that raise fundamental questions about the appropriate role of government generate what might be called 'stop and go' politics, long periods of gestation where partisan and ideological conflict invoke familiar symbols of legitimacy for and against state action.[15] Federal aid to education was one such issue in the 1950s and 1960s, similar in character to the 15-year battle over Medicare. Civil rights disputes are similar as well, struggles that awaken broad partisan position taking, passionate debate, and deeply held views that are seldom changed in the course of amassing support or opposition. In such issues, elections are crucial, mediated mandates from the electorate in which Presidents typically appeal for congressional approval in a direction supposedly dictated by the electorate.[16] There are few such issues at any one time and seldom has mental health – if ever – come on the national agenda in this form.

The more familiar policy disputes emerge from complex mixes of federal, state, and local action. They involve subsidy for some actions, constraint for others. They distribute burdens and benefits in ways that the ultimate payers and the payees need not confront each other directly. Colloquially known as pork barrel and regulatory politics, these familiar types of politics are central to the American pattern of policy-making in mental health.

One such form is the federal grant-in-aid, a subsidy from the national government to subnational units with strings attached. There are a vast number of categorical grants, with federal standards which state and local governments meet to some degree. Sometimes these lines of authority and standard-setting – as with the neighbourhood health centers of the 1960s – produce local units directly financed through federal programs but altered significantly to fit the political and social features of particular locales. These are examples of 'federal' programs that in fact have crucial local and (in the case of Community Mental Health Centers) state participation. At the other extreme are local policy domains – education or health care for the poor – where local action is significantly but indirectly shaped by federal rules, conventions, and financial incentives.

The sharing of and struggling over authority – both horizontally among the branches of government and vertically among the parts of American federalism – means that most governmental activity involves exceedingly complex bargaining among the component parts of each policy arena. This complexity is considerably increased by the many agencies and jurisdictions, all with overlapping responsibility but differing features. Legal arrangements, programs, and political settings vary immensely among the 50 states, 3,000 countries, and tens of thousands of local governments and special districts.[17]

But, for all the complexity, there is a simplicity about the strategies such fragmentation engenders. For those in the world of mental health services, as in many occupational spheres, there is a large gap between resources sought (needed) and those available. When single responsible authorities determine budgetary availability, persuasion, pressure, and the demonstration of opportunity costs make sense as tactics for a strategy of expansion. Where fragmentation is structural and continuing, the obvious incentive is different. It is to 'externalize' the costs to other jurisdictions and to 'internalize' administrative responsibility. Externalizing costs and internalizing benefits is a shorthand way of describing such political efforts. From the standpoint of state hospitals and local community mental health centres, federal funding illustrates the externalization of costs. The plea for flexibility and administrative authority at the state and local level expresses the continued concern for disconnecting direct finance from control of the administration of subnational programs. This pattern, dubbed the 'social pork barrel' by David Stockman, is evident in a wide variety of federal subsidy programs. Another way to characterize the pattern is to emphasize the per capita stakes of those on the finance and service sides of program bargaining. Local programs treat funding by state or federal sources as crucial parts of their financing; they have concentrated stakes in increasing those funds or avoiding losing them. Federal or state tax payers (and the budget officers who speak for their interest) have broadly diffused stakes in such programs. The per capita outlays of the entire mental health budget of the United States is dwarfed by the major spending programs in defence, conventional health services, and social security pensions. (For illustrative purposes, divide the 1980 outlays of $20 billion by a population of 200 million; contrast these per capita outlays of $100 with the substantial stakes of community mental health centres in federal contributions to their budgets). In this sense, fragmentation is part of the 'imbalanced political market' for social policies.[18]

There is an interesting twist to this same logic when one considers the reaction of local communities to mental patients displaced into their areas. In such instances, the general aim of deinstitutionalization — the benefits of which are averaged over the entire jurisdiction — produces concentrated 'losses' for the communities in which discharged patients locate themselves. Such arrangements conform to what Jack Pitney has called 'bile barrel' politics, the logical converse of pork barrel politics.[19] Where burdens are concentrated and benefits dispersed, no one should be surprised by the determined resistance of the concentrated losers, the communities most affected. Looked at this way, the pork barrel model makes sense of persistent postwar efforts to extend federal financing of mental health without creating local federal offices of mental health; the distribution of concentrated benefits and the dispersion of financial costs invite co-operation. But the same logic also explains why budget officials are wary of such arrangements. On the other hand, bile barrel politics makes understandable how it is that broad approval of politics like treatment 'in the community' is perfectly compatible with militant hostility to efforts to locate dischargees in particular communities. The same political logic, of course, extends to many other instances of threatening locations — prisons, toxic waste dumps, housing for the poor, and the like.[20]

Public vs private responsibility

Proposition three: *The politics of mental health are shaped, as well, by national understandings of what constitutes private and public responsibilities.*

In this respect, the long struggle over whether there is a federal responsibility for the provision and finance of personal health services has worked out differently in mental health.

For some 50 years in the United States there have been recurrent battles – fought with armies of pressure groups and the most compelling symbols of political legitimacy – over various forms of national health insurance. The alternatives regularly reviewed are repetitive: the theory of social insurance, with universal entitlement financed from a variety of sources versus the notion that most Americans can find their health insurance in the market and that government – local first, state second, and federal authorities third – is a last resort for those who are or will be destitute. The place of mental hospitals in this traditional struggle is anomalous; the care of the institutionalized mentally ill has been long regarded as a special state responsibility.[21] Within the political arena, the attack on the state mental hospitals was an example of the 'possible' set in opposition to the 'actual'. The hope was that local networks of mental health centres would some day supply the care for formerly institutionalized patients – and others – but never was the community mental health movement a major part of the broader battle over national health insurance, Medicare, and Medicaid.

Indeed, the major federal finance programs in health – Medicare and Medicaid – have been exceedingly wary of mental health services. For years, mental health services for the 22 to 64 age-group were not financed by Medicaid. And Medicare's psychiatric benefits – outside the hospital – have been derisory, $250/year. No wonder that innovative professionals in mental health have found themselves cut out from the major federal finance programs in medical care. In these respects, the two worlds of health care have been very differently conceptualized: one drawing from clear public responsibility – in both state and local jurisdictions – for the seriously mentally ill, with analogies to local public school districts responsible for all the 'eligible' students within an area. No one doubts that states have responsibility for public mental hospitals, though many argue about who should be treated and who should pay. The other tradition – in either the social insurance or the welfare form – has drawn more from the history of insurance, always wary of ill-defined conditions the budget implications of which are hard to estimate. The insurance tradition, wary of mental health, was also more congenially adapted to a national government perspective. No one, for instance, ever proposed that Medicare be financed and administered by the states and localities as in the case of community mental health centres.

For policy changes like Medicare, broad national consensus is required, but may not be sufficient for action. No such broad consensus existed – or exists –

regarding the care of the mentally ill. Within the professional community, there may be agreement on innovative modalities. But that agreement is not reflected in mass attention, supportive sentiment, or a willingness of governmental actors to place mental health finance prominently on the national agenda. What had once been a largely invisible world of mental hospitals, private suffering, and professional services now appears in local communities as homelessness, strange persons in public, and bewilderment about who is responsible for whom. In such a context, no wonder that those preoccupied with the mentally ill feel so frustrated with the politics of fiscal restraint in all the industrial democracies (see close of this chapter).

Role of the courts

Proposition four: *The courts play a special role in the politics of mental health.*

American courts have in the past two decades importantly shaped mental health practices. Our emphasis will not be on the string of cases and particularly important institutional examples, but rather on the place of court litigation in the political arena of mental health.

The connection between involuntary commitment and the protection of civil liberties is perhaps the most familiar topic in this broad area. Just as the ACLU (American Civil Liberties Union) has taken the protection of speech as one of its cherished objectives, so have legal reform groups seized on the protection of the mentally ill as worthy of special effort. And, in this latter area, there has been a close link between the broad discrediting of the state mental hospital and the penchant of litigious legal reformers for restricting the grounds on which the mentally disturbed can be involuntarily restrained. The twin tests of modern commitment procedures are the threat of harm to others or to oneself. In the absence of such threats, no one is justified in legally restricting the liberty of the ostensibly disturbed. We are unsure of how universal the practice of protecting the mentally ill from voluntary confinement – absent the threats cited above – really is. But we are quite sure that litigation in the United States has sharply affected the balance of interests over involuntary confinement.

The second area of interest is courts and institutional reform, legal intervention that affects the behaviour of mental institutions, particularly state hospitals. Since the widely noted Wyatt v. Stichney decision in 1971, there has been an explosion in legal challenges to conditions in large-scale institutions for the mentally ill and mentally retarded. At least three strands are worth noting. One is the set of challenges to the resources made available to mental institutions, the familiar argument that minimal standards of capacity are necessary before an institution can be regarded as acceptable. This is a common stage in public regulation generally, with professionals arguing about what would be required before a decent institution could open its doors or what would be the most obvious grounds for closing an institution. A second approach emphasizes outcomes, or the results of institutional 'treatment'. Here the criterion of evaluation was not solely whether an institution had the requisite inputs, but whether its performance 'helped' patients, or, at the least, did not produce retrogression. The Supreme Court is said[22] to have been somewhat ambivalent in support of this interpretation. But there is no question that the standard of performance competed with those of minimal inputs in the judicial evaluation of mental institutions. The third approach, one closely tied to the deinstitutionalization movement, sought to change the site of services to the mentally ill. The aim was to certify the community as the sole location where constitutionally adequate treatment was possible. This view held that constitutionally adequate care could not be provided in large scale mental institutions, a position symbolized in the famous Pennhurst decision of 1977.[23]

This is but the roughest of summaries of the complex role of the American judiciary in the recent history of mental health policies and programs. We want to raise here three issues without claiming to go beyond the stage of highlighting a topic. First, it is worth noting that the arena of courts – rather than legislatures – puts the administrators of large-scale institutions in a less advantaged political position. It is not difficult to find highly skilled legal advocates whose relatively superior capacity to attack both existing conditions and the rationales of operational managers is obvious. Both the input and performance measures of large-scale institutions can be articulated in such a way that, for the court, the question is seemingly simple: if these measures cannot be satisfied, is incarceration warranted? The distributional particular consequences of such a decision are before courts. But the local communities are not parties to a decision about whether an institution satisfies minimal standards set by courts. It is easy to imagine institutional managers overwhelmed by demands made upon them for which the relevant resources – drawn from other parts of the political order – are simply not available. The third standard – the constitutional inadequacy of large-scale institutionalization itself – makes moot the issue of resources. And it is fair to say that, in the 1980s the phenomenon of homelessness – and the prominent place of discharged mental patients among the homeless – generated some counter-reaction. The American Psychiatric Association has drafted a somewhat less strict definition of commitability – substituting the risk of substantial deterioration for the more demanding standard of dangerousness to oneself and others. Whatever the state of judicial opinion, it is clear that innovative approaches to mental health will be subject to judicial scrutiny to a degree that seems quite remarkable in the context of international comparison.

This conclusion mirrors quite closely the conventional interpretation of the role of courts in the world of American mental health over the past 30 years. There are, of course, other interpretations possible. The very fragmentation of authority in American politics opens up quite diverse strategies to interested parties. One such strategy is the use of court directives to further the purposes of hospital administrators who were after all, parties to the consent decrees of the 1970s. On this interpretation, judicial activism might be seen in part as the desirable course for beleagured administrators, actors managing institutions for scorned patients, which had a low priority on the budgetary agendas of state politics. For such administrators litigation directed against the conditions of their hospitals might – implicitly or explicitly but not publicly – have been welcome. The meaning of consent decrees – illustrated by the Wyatt v. Stickney and Willowbrook instances – would differ greatly from the interpretation above. The very advantages of the legal critics would serve the masked aims of such administrative reformers. Court action would prompt outcomes which the normal politics of state budgeting had blocked; the details of the consent decrees would constitute pressures on administrative implementation that ordinary politics could not have been relied upon to deliver. Caution is needed about the conventional understanding of the resistant administrator compelled to accept court action against his or her will.[24]

Proposition five: *The broader political economy of the American welfare state has crucially constrained the options in all arenas of American social policy, including mental health.*

America's reactions to stagflation in the 1970s and the budget deficits of the 1980s dominated domestic social policy politics. It is true that macroeconomic trends – the inflation of the Viet Nam years and the stagflation that worsened after the oil crisis of 1973–74 – set the direction of policy responses but did not determine their particular shape. Whatever degree of spending restraint was called for, American politics generated a widespread sense of crisis in social policy. The claim of a crisis meant, for example, that national health insurance would become progressively unthinkable as the low growth of the economy reduced forecasted revenues and the tax cuts of 1981, coupled with the arms build-up of the Carter–Reagan years, produced very large federal deficits. Deficits, a large and growing defence budget, and the political unwillingness to raise taxes substantially has put all of medical care – and its mental health component – in a paralytic vice. Only policy proposals that promise reductions in federal expenditures – like the heralded Diagnostic Related Groups innovation in Medicare hospital reimbursement (1983) – easily get on the agenda of active discussion. Otherwise, social policy energy has largely concentrated on protecting current programs from further budget cutbacks. And the Gramm–Rudman–Hollings legislation of 1985 institutionalized the politics of constraint, making large-scale programmatic innovation practically unthinkable.

This broader context of imprisonment will not easily change. No amount of innovation in a social policy arena will command wide audiences without evidence of fiscal saving or, at the least, no great federal financial commitments. The key to change here is not developments within particular policy areas, however innovative and promising, but in the broader political economy of the country. Increased economic growth or the increased willingness to raise taxes – either or both – are the keys to a changed context for the implementation of mental health innovations. It may be that within large programs – in medical care, housing, and education – there are margins for adjustment that recognize the nonmedical aspects of the care of the mentally ill. But we leave that discussion to another time. Our point here is that the political–economic setting – as illustrated in the five broad generalizations offered above – constrains mental health to a degree that is worthy of special emphasis.

Conclusion

The central theme of this chapter has been the impact of American political arrangements on the difficulties in implementing innovative mental health programs on which there is substantial and positive professional consensus. Two developments in mental health politics have prompted extensive commentary in recent decades. One is the conjunction of the rapid reduction in the numbers of the mentally ill hospitalized in state institutions and the failure of the budgets of state hospitals to fall proportionately. The other is the large gap between the acknowledged difficulties of discharged patients and the dream of community care that would take up where state hospitals had supposedly failed so completely. Does a focus on American political arrangements particularly – and political analysis of the distribution of gains and losses generally – offer any distinctive illumination?

The finding that the budgets of mental hospitals did not fall in proportion to their declining role in the treatment of the mentally ill is not surprising to the political analyst. Whenever the gains of change fall on one party and the losses on another – in the United States, Britain, or any other setting – losers will resist even if the marginal gains of expenditure elsewhere are greater. The effort to keep hospital budgets from falling was utterly predictable. It has proven very difficult to shift budgets away from state mental hospitals to community alternatives. Part of the reason is jurisdictional, the fact that different authorities administer programs in and outside mental hospitals; that of course is true for Britain as well and helps to explain why the British authors of chapters in this book emphasize the resistance to moving resources from one sector to produce greater gains in another. But American fragmentation makes more obvious what is evident everywhere. With multiple authorities in mental health – as elsewhere – the political logic of agreement on the benefits of care outside institutions is perfectly compatible with determined resistance to giving up one's budget to make reform easier. Moreover, state mental hospitals are large employers in their communities; bed closings and layoffs impose concentrated losses which geographically based state representatives predictably resist even if the same resources could be, according to the professionals, better spent elsewhere.

The mismatches between social need and spending patterns are striking. During the 1965–75 decade, spending for mental health increased sharply; the fragmented 'pork barrels' of mental health floated, so to speak, on a rising tide. But adverse economic conditions, itself a cause of increased mental distress, had the predicted impact on the funding of services. Whereas spending for major mental health facilities grew in the first half of the 1970s at an average annual rate of 12%, the share of GNP devoted to mental health fell 28% between 1977 and 1980. All the fragments of American mental health funding experienced budget pressures; the context of budget famine made reallocation difficult at the very time economic distress increased the need for it. Medicaid, now the largest single source of funds for mental health care, allocates some two-thirds of its mental health budget for institutional services and has extraordinarily low rates of payment for outpatient care. Nonetheless, state Medicaid officials fear more generous funding of outpatient care will add to its outlays without substituting for the more expensive institutional services. And, since no state or federal official is responsible for the overall allocation, the results of mismatch can continue almost indefinitely.

The reality of mismatch is obvious in the disappointing features of deinstitutionalization. On the one hand, the deinstitutionalization movement has been extraordinarily powerful, literally transforming the site of care for the severely mentally ill. But few express satisfaction with the responses within communities to the discharged patients. The growth and diversification of mental health services, financed substantially by federal categorical programs, did not match the transparent needs of discharged patients. The funds required to support these patients in community settings were not forthcoming; the patients themselves had no vouchers – representing savings from foregone institutional care – for the new services required. And the service system, financed by multiple sources, was difficult for patients to use, criticized as wasteful, and labelled as extraordinarily complex.[25] Fragmentation, stagflation, and budget deficits constituted a brew in the 1980s decidedly unhealthy for the implementation of innovative programs in the care and financing of the chronically mentally ill.

The impact of recent political change is likely to be quite limited in the world of mental health. The scope of proposition five above – the political paralysis over deficits, tax increases, and the spending for defence, social security, and Medicare/Medicaid – is very broad. Only the most favoured groups in society will find their needs on the agenda of public expansion. In that competition the needs of children and health concerns over catastrophic expenses (particularly for the elderly and employed adults) command far greater public appeal than the problems of the mentally ill. Straightened circumstances for federal budgets including those for the mentally ill will be with us as far as the eye can see.

For historians of American health policy, the crucial legacy of the Reagan administration will not be official policies towards the mentally ill, but the creation of an environment in which large-scale innovation for the socially disfavoured is today practically unthinkable. That environmental legacy was shaped by the early years of the Reagan presidency, the tax cuts of 1981, the build-up of defence expenditures throughout the first term, and the creation of budget deficits that 'voodoo' economics were allegedly to cure. There are no fiscal dividends to allocate to the disfavoured. And, as a result, the problems of implementing innovative programs in mental health will largely remain in the fragmented world of mental health. In that world, only the most determined and entrepreneurial of professional leaders will be able to force reallocation of resources

Research for this paper was supported, in part, by a grant to the Institution for Social and Policy Studies and Professor Marmor from the Henry J. Kaiser Family Foundation of Menlo Park, California. A revised version of this chapter appeared in the *Journal of Health Politics, Policy and Law*, 1989, **14**, No. 3. Fall.

Notes

1. National Institute of Mental Health, *Mental Health US* (ADM) 85-1378. (Washington, DC: US Government Printing Office), p. 99.
2. As Note 1.
3. This phenomenon, as the chapters by Carrier and Yellowlees show, is true of Britain as well, suggesting that the fate of innovative programs is worsened in conditions of budget austerity, conditions that have applied in both the United States and Great Britain since stagflation developed after the oil-price explosion of 1973–74.
4. Mary Lou Cooper, *Private Health Insurance Benefits for Alcoholism, Drug Abuse, and Mental Illness*, Intergovernmental Health Policy Project, (Washington, DC: George Washington University, July 1979), p. 3.
5. *Task Panel Reports Submitted to the President's Commission on Mental Health*, v. 2, app. (Washington, DC: US Government Printing Office, 1978), pp. 448–450.
6. See Carrier's chapter (9) in this Volume, of the difficulties created by the separation of payment to professional health workers like physicians (out of the NHS budget) from the payment to psychiatric social workers and other community care givers (out of local authority budgets) in Britain.
7. The similarity to British problems is striking and reported well in both the Yellowlees and the Carrier chapters in this Volume.
8. Morton Kramer, Mental Disorders as a Public Health Problem, presented at Preventive Medicine and Public Health Conference, The Johns Hopkins University School of Hygiene and Public Health, Baltimore, Maryland, April 30, 1982. See also *Task Panel Reports*, p. 85.
9. As Note 8, p. 89.
10. For a thoughtful treatment of the gap between American political beliefs and practice,

see Samuel P. Huntington, *American Politics: The Promise of Disharmony* (Harvard University Press: Cambridge, MA, 1981).

11. See, for example, Jameson W. Doig & Erwin C. Hargrove (eds), *Leadership and Innovation: A Bibliographical Perspective on Entrepreneurs in Government* (Baltimore, MD: The Johns Hopkins University Press, 1987), especially T. R. Marmor, Public Management: Wilbur Cohen and Robert Ball (pp. 246–281). For a more general discussion of the difficulty of implementing innovative programs within the world of American politics, see T. R. Marmor and A. Dunham, Political Science and Health Services Administration, in T. R. Marmor, *Political Analysis and American Medical Care* (New York: Cambridge University Press, 1983) pp. 5–44.

12. The problems of implementation for American political analysis is developed at length in Judith Feder, John Holahan, and Theodore Marmor (eds) *National Health Insurance: Conflicting Goals and Policy Choices* (Washington, DC: The Urban Institute, 1980).

13. This sketch of British concentration of authority may seem in conflict with the chapters by Yellowlees and Carrier, both of which emphasize how difficult it has been to implement allegedly agreed-upon reforms of community services for those discharged from mental hospitals. But what we have argued here suggests not that implementation will be easy in Britain but that it will be even more difficult in a fragmented polity like that of the United States. The constrained budget environment of both countries has reduced the chances for implementation of any innovative programs requiring new public funds; this common feature should not obscure the relatively greater fragmentation in the United States. Or, put another way, had our British colleagues been analyzing the United States, they would have been startled by the even greater problems of co-ordination here.

14. Gerald N. Grob, *Mental Illness and American Society, 1875–1940* (Princeton University Press: Princeton, NJ, 1983).

15. Nelson Polsby, *Political Innovation in America: The Politics of Policy Initiation* (New Haven: Yale University Press, 1984).

16. See, for example, T. R. Marmor, *The Politics of Medicare* (Aldine: Chicago, 1973), Chapter 6.

17. Jerry L. Mashaw & Susan Rose Ackerman, Federalism and Regulation, in Eads and Fix (eds.) *Reagan's Regulatory Strategy III*, (Washington, DC: Urban Institute Press, 1985), pp. 111–45.

18. Theodore R. Marmor, Donald A. Wittman & Thomas C. Heagy, The Politics of Medical Inflation, in Marmor, *Political Analysis*, pp. 61–75.

19. John J. Pitney, Bile Barrel Politics: Siting Unwanted Facilities *Journal of Policy Analysis and Management* 3 (Spring) 1984, pp. 446–448.

20. Timothy J. Sullivan, *Resolving Development Disputes Through Negotiation* (Plenum Press: New York and London, 1984).

21. Grob, *Mental Illness*, and Henry A. Foley & Steven S. Sharfstein, *Madness in Government: Who Cares for the Mentally Ill.* (American Psychiatric Press: Washington, DC, 1983) pp. 103–5.

22. Conversation with Robert Burt, Professor of Law at Yale University, October 21, 1986.

23. Halderman v. Pennhurst State School & Hospital 446 F. Supp. 1295 (E. D. Pa. 1977).

For details and analysis of this important and complicated case's history, see Robert Burt, Pennhurst: A Parable, in Robert H. Mnookin (ed.) *In the Interest of Children: Advocacy, Law Reform and Public Policy* (New York: W. H. Freeman, 1985), pp. 266–363.

24. I have benefited here, as elsewhere, from the thoughtful observations of Professor Robert Burt, my friend and colleague who has advanced some of these views in his article on the Pennhurst case cited in Note 23.

25. Steven S. Sharfstein, Medical Cutbacks and Block Grants: Crisis or Opportunity for Community Health? *American Journal of Psychiatry*, **139**, No. 4 (April, 1982, p. 466).

11

Mental health care in continental Europe: medley or mosaic?

Norman Sartorius

Is there a European model of mental health care? Is the similarity among the ideals, tenets, and organizational forms of mental health services in continental Europe sufficient to constitute a unity, a mosaic which, although composed of a multitude of constituents, presents a coherent, recognizable image with which one can compare service systems used in other parts of the world? Or, are there so many differences among the European countries that it is foolish to even attempt a comparison of, say, the system of services in the USA with that in 'Europe'?

To deal with this question three others have to be answered first:

1. Are there indicators (such as, for example, the proportion of people with a disease who benefit from a service) which can be used to describe the function of a mental health service system in a valid and parsimonious way? Are those who study service systems and describe them willing to use such indicators in a uniform way?

2. Is there information which is necessary to describe the mental health service systems? Does the central statistical office, for example, have access to information about the treatment of the mentally ill provided by psychiatrists in private practice? Are the differences among countries in the amount of such information, its credibility, ease of access and comprehensiveness of coverage so significant that no comparison can be made?

3. What is the most reasonable unit of counting, in terms of time and coverage? Is there any point in using cross-sectional census data or should these only be examined if they can be compared with similar data

obtained for other points in time? is it reasonable to consider data for a country as a whole[1] or is it necessary to examine data for much smaller administrative (e.g. district) or sociocultural (e.g. national) groups?

This paper will first examine these three questions, then present some data about the situation in Europe and end by an attempt to summarize common trends in service development.

Indicators of mental health care

Mental health programs differ from plans for psychiatric services. The latter deal with ways and means of developing services for the mentally ill and, in some settings, for their families. Mental health programs are broader: they deal not only with the care of the mentally ill but also with public health action necessary to prevent mental illness, with social measures necessary to promote the value of mental health, and with the contribution which mental health disciplines – including psychiatry and behavioural sciences such as psychology and anthropology – can make to the performance of the general health services and to overall socioeconomic development (Sartorius & Harding, 1983; WHO, 1981). This part of the paper will deal with indicators used in the planning, functioning and evaluation of services for the mentally ill and not with those describing other components of mental health programs (e.g. the effectiveness of mental health education campaigns).

There is little agreement among decision-makers, mental health experts, statisticians, epidemiologists and others involved in the provision of services for the mentally ill about which indicators should be used in the description of services for the mentally ill. As a consequence, it is very difficult to find two countries – and more recently even two states within countries with a federal system – which present data about their mental health services in similar ways.

Even when apparently similar indicators are used, their definition is different. A 'psychiatric bed' will, in the report of one country, refer exclusively to beds in public mental hospitals; in others, beds in private psychiatric institutions are also counted. Beds in sheltered accommodation (e.g. hostels, night hospitals, etc) are sometimes included or reported separately or not at all. Nursing home beds – which are becoming more and more important in the system of services for the mentally ill – are often not reported as psychiatric beds even though many of the inmates suffer from mental illness. In some European countries health statistics include no information about facilities managed by other social service systems (e.g. facilities for the mentally ill and impaired run by the Ministry of Social Welfare or Education). Information about personnel or facilities administered by, say, religious institutions are often omitted entirely. There are settings in which some parts of a system such as those set up by a charity may provide reports to the government while others do not, for historical or unknown reasons. The figures obtained thus represent different parts of the total of services in various countries and can at best be used as rough estimates.

Comparison within the same country or province over time is equally risky: changes in the organization of services (e.g. complete or partial separation between neurology and psychiatry) often render figures incomparable. Sometimes the changes in service structure are accompanied by appropriate changes in information systems; when this does not happen 'inexplicable' trends appear in the data. Changes in parts of the statistical machinery, e.g. replacement of one classification system by a new one are yet another of the many developments that can make time series analyses meaningless.

Information available in European countries

Differences between countries in terms of effort invested to produce information and preserve it are much smaller than differences in the definition of indicators. Remarkable quantities of data are collected even in countries in which resources for health care are scarce and in which the probability that significant changes will occur because of indications contained in the data is low or nonexistent. Someone compared the ever-growing appetite for data to the mythical simpleton who saw that potatoes get softer when boiled longer and hoped that the same would happen if he boiled eggs longer: since small amounts of well-selected information made it easier to reach reasonable conclusions, there is a notion that more data would make conclusions even better and easier to reach. The increasing yen for data could of course have a variety of other explanations, including the inertia of administrations who tend to continue the collection of data long after the purpose of collecting them has been forgotten; the growing number of public health decision-makers appointed to their position by simple transfer from clinical work and applying rules governing small-scale clinical studies to national, routine statistics; the use of the size of the data collection systems as an argument for power claims and advancement in political careers; and the use of the 'need to collect more data' as the reason to avoid making a decision.

Technological advances in data management have also contributed to the appetite for data collection but seem to have little or no effect on either the quality of statistical reports or on the delay in their publication. In spite of a vast expansion of the potential of statistical systems, the quality and timeliness of reports as well as the willingness to use the results of their analysis have declined.

Trends towards decentralization and increasing independence of federal states have also decreased the capacity of central statistical offices to obtain and publish anything but the most banal data. The argument that data can be best used by those closest to their source has been used not only to justify the development of mechanisms to transmit data to the periphery, but also to stop providing data to central authorities. Time series have therefore been broken in a number of countries. Unfortunately the weakening of central statistical offices has not resulted in strengthening of the periphery; on the contrary, the weakness of the centre has meant a weakening of methodological assistance, lack of leadership and of external pressure to continue collecting data and control their quality.

Units of analysis

There is little agreement, also, on which units of analysis – in terms of time period and population coverage – are best to describe mental health care. There are numerous reasons for this discord. One lies in the nature of mental disorders which often have an insidious onset, an ill defined midpoint and a clinical course which varies from person to person and from one time to the next. Another is the dependence of the severity of the impairment caused by illness and of subsequent disability on a variety of sociocultural factors. Political necessity (e.g. the use of longer time periods to indicate the insignificance of a particularly alarming development), practical difficulties (e.g. limitation of time series because of service changes) and traditions prevalent in a country or region further contribute to the difficulty of agreeing on the most convenient units of analysis.

Similar discord is also present in discussions about the size of population or territory that should be used to describe the service system. The previous insistence on presenting data for a country as a whole has recently been criticized because a large assembly of data can hide trends and special situations. The presentation of data for a large geographically defined area has also been criticized because such areas often contain markedly different districts, and because of the increasing number of instances in which care is provided by organizations located outside the area (e.g. industrial medical services).

Sociocultural differences have been recognized as an important determinant of mental disorder, influencing its occurrence, course and outcome: the consequence was an attempt to construct units of statistical and epidemiological analysis for subgroups of populations living in the same geographical area (e.g. the French-speaking inhabitants of Brussels). The difficulty in this otherwise commendable approach is that the amount of sociocultural identification is often difficult to assess: most of the members of the two or more socioculturally defined groups living next to each other tend to resemble one another more than their more distinguishable forebears. Real differences that may have existed among groups and usually disappear over time unless there are (usually political) reasons to maintain and promote differences. If this is the case, the result can be, and often is, a wasteful search for nonexistent differences in health states and the predominantly nonscientific use of findings. So, for example, intensive research into social moves and disease prevalence in migrant groups is often motivated by the wish to demonstrate that migrants are different and spend more than an

Table 11.1. *Changes in number of beds for the treatment of patients with psychiatric disorders.*

	1972	1982
Psychiatric hospitals	202	96
Psychiatric units in general hospital	408	615
Number of beds in psychiatric units	24,971	37,398
Percentage of total number of psychiatric beds in psychiatric units:	6	10
Mental hospital beds per 1000 inhabitants in:		
Yugoslavia	0·8	0·8
Ireland	5·8	4·2

appropriate share of health care resources, and should therefore be sent back to their country of origin. Other situations in which national or ethnic rivalry in a country are present provide numerous examples of this type of misleading use of research efforts and of data about health.

A sample of European data

In spite of the above difficulties it is possible to use data obtained in European countries provided that (a) these are understood as estimates rather than as exact measurements; (b) that they are compared (and corrected) with other sources of knowledge about the countries (e.g. ethnographical or literary descriptions); (c) that they are not used as proof that certain interventions have or have not led directly to their change.[2]

Used in this way, the analysis of even the (somewhat flawed) data that can be obtained from countries in Europe indicates significant changes in European mental health services over the past few decades. This is well illustrated by data from recent publications (Breemer ter Stege & Gittelman, 1987; WHO, 1987; Mangen, 1985) and from a recent WHO survey (Freeman *et al.*, 1985) which showed the following.

1. The number of mental hospitals with more than 1000 beds has decreased in Europe over the last decade. A comparison of data from 21 countries (excluding France, USSR and the Federal Republic of Germany which did not provide data in time for inclusion in this analysis) showed that the total number of hospitals with more than 1000 beds fell from 202 to 96. There was a slight increase in the average size of hospitals with under 1000 beds in 13 countries (Table 11.1).

2. Over the past decade the number of psychiatric units in general hospitals has increased. Comparisons could be made in 17 countries. The total number of such units has grown from 408 to 615 with a corresponding

Table 11.2. *Mental health personnel:*
(a) *Numbers of psychiatrists per 100,000 population.*

Belgium	(1984)	12·7
Denmark	(1982)	8·3
France	(1980)	5·1
F.R. Germany	(1982)	8·3
Ireland	(1981)	5·3
Italy	(1981)	2·1
Luxembourg	(1977)	6·6
The Netherlands	(1982)	6·1
United Kingdom	(1981)	7·6

(b) *Numbers of psychologists per psychiatrist.*

1972	1982
0·3	0·59

(c) *Numbers of nurses with training in psychiatry per psychiatrist.*

Ireland	23·3
Malta	31·9
Czechoslovakia	0·3
Greece	0·4

increase of beds in those units from 24,971 to 37,398. These beds, however, represented only 6% of all psychiatric beds in 1972 and only 10% of all beds in 1982.

3. The number of beds in mental hospitals could be compared in 28 countries. In 1972 the lowest number of beds was in Yugoslavia (0·8 per 1,000) and the highest in Ireland (5·8 per 1,000). By 1982, the number of beds per 1,000 population had fallen in 15 countries and risen in 5, but the increases were minimal.

4. Another indicator concerns the length of stay, which can be expressed as the number of admissions per psychiatric bed. In 1982, variations within Europe were enormous. In Malta and the Netherlands the number of admissions per bed was 1·03 and 1·05 respectively. In Iceland and Hungary at the other end of the scale the number of admissions per bed was 9·57 and 6·52 respectively.

5. The number of outpatient contacts per 100,000 inhabitants per year varied considerably between countries, from 1450 in Ireland to 12,983 in Czechoslovakia.

6. The number of psychiatrists per 100,000 inhabitants showed up to a five-fold difference among countries, being 2·3 in Malta, 10 in Belgium, and 12·7 in Iceland (Table 11.2).

The number of psychologists was growing faster than the numbers of psychiatrists. In the 17 countries in which a comparison was possible the number of psychologists per psychiatrist doubled from 0·3 in 1972 to 0·6 in 1982. The highest number of psychologists employed in mental health services in Europe today is in Norway (0·93 per psychiatrist). The differences among countries in number of psychiatric nurses are even larger: in Ireland and Malta the ratio is 23·3 and 31·9 nurses per psychiatrist while in Czechoslovakia and Greece the ratio is 0·3 and 0·4 nurses per psychiatrist.

Trends affecting mental health care in Europe
These findings have to be examined in the broader context of changes and trends in European mental health services. They include the following:

Decentralization of health services
In most European countries there is a trend towards a policy of geographical decentralization of services. Psychiatric services are increasingly often being established in areas distant from the capital. Improved communications and transport to peripheral parts of the country, better schooling and universal access to material (and cultural) goods have acted as a powerful factor in the decisions of younger staff to move to peripheral units. By and large, the quality of care did not decrease in the decentralized system, and a number of excellent peripheral services have sprung up in many countries.

There is considerable variation between European countries (and among states in countries with a federal structure) in the amount of administrative autonomy given to the peripheral services. Usually this autonomy depends less on legal provisions and more on the attitude and style of administration of the local authorities than on the personality of the psychiatrist who heads the service.

There has also been an extensive 'ideological' decentralization of health care. While previously there was both an expectation of leadership and an acceptance of the principles of health care stated by the central authority with the technical blessing of the university department of psychiatry in the capital, there is now a clear trend towards increased independence in most European countries' peripheral services.

Growth of self-help movements
In a considerable number of countries in Europe, self-help movements have become an important factor in psychiatric care. Some of them are organizations of patients such as Depressives Anonymous, others involve parents or relatives of schizophrenics or other types of patients. The self-help groups vary and seem to

fall neatly into three groups: those that act as an extension of the psychiatric service and abide by the rules and instructions given by that service; those which are established in opposition to the psychiatric service and actively militate against individual psychiatrists, the profession and the service as a whole; and finally those that are independent but willing to negotiate with psychiatric services about various issues and accept some advice and guidance. Self-help movements flourish in the North: in the South of Europe they are much less well developed and accepted only with reluctance.

The efficiency drive

In several European countries the cost of care has gone up so quickly and so much that drastic measures have been taken to stem further cost explosion. In some instances (e.g. the United Kingdom) it has been recommended that professional administrators (regardless of how much they know about psychiatry) become managers of psychiatric services at community and district levels. In other countries, a significant amount of administrative control has been introduced, often entailing considerable expense and causing delays and dissatisfaction within the service and in the population services. Cost reduction schemes are being tried out in a number of countries; their life is usually short and they often disappear or get replaced by new schemes even before they have been fully assessed and described. The entry of private international hospital chains into European countries has also contributed to the attention given to economy of service provision and to the rationalization of expenditures in the public sector (e.g. in Switzerland).

Emphasis on quality assurance

A most welcome trend in a number of European countries has been the growing emphasis on quality of care taking on a variety of forms, from peer review to establishment of special inspectorates (e.g. in the Netherlands) that monitor quality of care. New modalities such as special committees (involving medical personnel and others) to control quality of patient care, and multidisciplinary teams to analyse accidents in hospitals have come into existence and represent desirable innovations in the efforts to ensure minimal standards of care. The decrease in size of psychiatric facilities and the delegation of power to local authorities have both helped and hindered control of the quality of care in some countries. Helped, because those who control are more familiar with the situation and more aware of both constraints and possibilities. Hindered because independence from the central authority also meant that funds necessary to introduce innovations have to be found locally by reducing some other activity financed by the peripheral authority. Furthermore, local authorities do not always see the necessity for research which was earlier carried out as part of service; nor is it always easy to find ways of supporting work on matters which were traditionally carried out by the central administration of services to large populations (e.g. developing strategies to help patients with a rare disease or with an unusual combination of needs).

Reviews of mental health legislation

Legislation concerning the treatment of the mentally ill and the promotion of mental health has been revised in a number of European countries (for an account see, e.g. Mangen, 1985). In the new laws there is more emphasis on the protection of patients' human rights and individual responsibility. A regrettable consequence of the concern about confidentiality of data about patients was the disestablishment of several psychiatric registers in Europe (e.g. in the Federal Republic of Germany).

Emergence of new forms of psychiatric services

A variety of 'new' psychiatric services have come into existence. Some of them are the consequence of the search for 'a place under the sun' by professions rather than a result of a rational analysis of patients' needs and ways to satisfy them. Crisis intervention units, for example, have sprung up in a number of countries. A recent analysis demonstrated considerable differences in their structure and content of work (see Chapter by Katschnig & Konieczna, this volume) which are often new in name only (Cooper, 1979). The use of 'nonscientific' medicine and 'traditional healers' of different types from magnetizers and hand layers to herbalists and astrologers seems to be on the increase in most European countries. Exact figures are difficult to obtain for the total number of healers and for the number of patients visiting them. Anecdotal reports, however, indicate that the numbers of healers match or exceed the numbers of doctors trained in recognized medical schools. Patients seem to use the services of practitioners of 'soft medicine' and of those trained in medical schools.

Training in mental health care

The differences in style, duration and content of undergraduate and postgraduate training in psychiatry in Europe have, if anything, increased over the past decade (Lenz, 1984). Definitions of minimal training for psychiatrists and other mental health service staff differ widely. In some countries there are no examinations for mental health workers. In others there are examinations for several degrees which are extremely formalized. Differences between countries have rendered exchange of staff, fellowship programmes, and similar activities increasingly difficult.

Growth of 'new' professions

Recent years have seen the emergence of powerful interprofessional rivalries in the field of mental health. Psychologists have become much more numerous, contend for the 'mental health dollar' and request legislative procedures that would enable them to practise not only psychiatry but also 'behavioural medicine'. Other professions have also grown in numbers, request independence and contend for their share in the treatment of disease. General practitioners and specialists in internal medicine who had brief training in psychology or psychiatry, psychiatric social workers, 'defectologists', speech therapists and a variety of other professions have increased in numbers: in contrast, psychiatric nursing has had a significant drop in the number of entrants. This is partly due to the decrease in the number of psychiatric hospitals (and thus posts); partly to the increasing complexity and length of basic and post-basic nursing training which makes many candidates opt for medicine or other health professions with more prestige than nursing.

Continuing lack of administrative coordination

A continuing problem on the European mental health scene is the lack of coordination between the various social service sectors involved in care for the mentally ill and impaired. In some countries (e.g. the Netherlands), co-ordinating committees involving representatives of different sectors have been set up with beneficial effects; in others parliamentary commissions have been established to examine mental health care and recommend changes (e.g. in the Federal Republic of Germany). Most European countries, however, have not yet acted to reduce overlap and render activities of the different sectors more logical, coherent and useful. Programs for alcohol and drug-related health problems and those for mental retardation illustrate this tendency particularly well. Although usually handled by mental health services those activities are in some countries taken out of the health system altogether and are being managed by the Ministry of Interior, Social Welfare, or other bodies.

Simplification of psychiatric treatment and rehabilitation techniques

Techniques for use in the field of mental health care have been exposed to serious scrutiny and some (such as ECT) are disappearing from use in services in some countries (e.g. in Switzerland). There has been a conscious and intensive effort to simplify psychiatric techniques and make it possible for general practitioners and other health staff to deal with mental disorders in a competent way. Weekend courses on the management of depression (and similar training activities) for general practitioners enjoy considerable popularity. Numerous manuals and instructions on ways to deal with a particular problem in oneself or in patients are being published and widely distributed among professionals and even among the lay public. The use of psychoanalysis and its appeal are by and large on the decline: there are, however, major differences between countries in this respect.

Conclusion

The question posed in the introduction to this paper can now be answered. Despite their differences, European countries show sufficient similarities in philosophy, trends and current forms of service provision to constitute a 'model' of mental health care. This model, is not vastly different from, say, the model of psychiatric care developed in Canada or Australia; the model is that of a developed, industrialized country.

This is not to say that industrialized countries do not differ in the organization of their psychiatric services. Differences *within* countries also exist and can be so important that they overshadow differences *between* countries. The services providing care in the north of Italy are more similar to those of its northern neighbours than to those in the south of the country. The provinces of Spain differ significantly from one another in culture, social development and health service models and so do the Länder of Germany, the départements of France and the communities of Belgium.

Data about European psychiatric services are not satisfactory. The definitions of indicators which would help in monitoring development and functioning of services are not generally accepted and the data available suffice at best to make educated guesses and estimations rather than detailed factual comparisons.

Particularly lacking are indicators of satisfaction with services, of those who provide them and of those who use them; indicators of changes in the quality of life of people in treatment; and indicators of psychosocial characteristics of various types of institutions for long-term care (e.g. nursing homes).

But even for indicators which have been used for a long time there are no standard and generally accepted definitions (e.g. on what constitutes a psychiatric bed or good outcome of treatment). In the few instances in which there are elements that would allow the uniform interpretation of an indicator (e.g. on the number of grand mal epileptics in a community) there are no data for populations over time.

There have been significant changes in European mental health services over the past few decades. These present rich material for study and call for methodological development which will make it possible to describe and assess innovations in service delivery so as to make it possible to disseminate those which were found to be valuable across Europe and to other parts of the world.

Notes:

1. This question may be particularly important in considering data from countries with a federal structure in which the constituent states or provinces of a country can differ vastly from each other.
2. The recent papers from Italy showing that there was a tendency towards reduction in

the numbers of psychiatric inpatient beds over many years prior to the Law 180, and the analyses showing that mental hospitals in the UK were reduced in size before the introduction of psychopharmacological treatments, are both examples of recent corrections of a fallacy in causal linkage.

References

Breemer ter Stege, C. & Gittelman, M. (1987). The Direction of Change in Western European Mental Health Care. In *Trends in Mental Health Care in Western Europe in the past 25 years. International Journal of Mental Health*, **16**, No. 1–2.

Cooper, J. E. (1979). Crisis Admission Units and Emergency Psychiatric Services. *Public Health in Europe*, **11**. World Health Organization, Regional Office for Europe, Copenhagen.

Freeman, H. L., Fryers, T. and Henderson, J. H. (1985). *Mental Health Services in Europe: 10 years on.* World Health Organization, Regional Office for Europe, Copenhagen.

Lenz, G. (1984). Postgraduate Training in Developing Countries. A Questionnaire Study by the WPA Secretariat. In (J. J. Lopéz-Ibor Aliño and G. Lenz, eds). *Training and Education in Psychiatry*, p. 284, Facultas, Vienna.

Mangen, S. P. (ed.) (1985). *Mental Health Care in the European Community*. Croom Helm, London, Sydney, Dover, New Hampshire.

Sartorius, N. & Harding, T. W. (1983). Issues in the evaluation of mental health care. In *Evaluation of Health Care*. (Holland, W. W., ed.), pp. 226–242. Oxford Medical Publications, Oxford, New York, Toronto.

World Health Organization (WHO) (1981). *Social Dimensions of Mental Health.* WHO: Geneva.

World Health Organization (WHO), Regional Office for Europe, Copenhagen (1987). Mental Health Services in Pilot Study Areas.

Section E: Administrative

Editors' commentary

Yellowlees, Klerman and Pardes draw from their considerable experience to indicate some of the many administrative hurdles that impede the dissemination of potentially useful innovations. Yellowlees indicates the need for start-up money to introduce new methods, and the need to win the hearts and minds of potential opponents who fear they might lose from the proposed change, in order to overcome their resistance or apathy. The Robert Wood Johnson Foundation's 9-Cities program is an outstanding attempt to overcome some barriers to the forging of effective community care for serious mental illness by providing seed money to centres once they have got their act together by producing an integrated authority to deliver such care. Though throwing money at a problem by itself cures little, appropriately contingent funds can be a powerful incentive for groups to co-operate and change.

There are limits to what can be achieved in an adverse political climate with even the most sophisticated wheeling and dealing. Pardes relates the sobering story of how the Mental Health Systems Act promising significant advances in mental health care delivery became law at the end of Carter's administration, only to be overturned a couple of months later as soon as Reagan became President.

Pardes draws some lessons from this experience. There is a need for more advocacy for people with mental illness, for programs to be based on solid data and regular evaluation with modesty without promising more than can be delivered, and for populations with different needs to be catered for differentially.

12

Administrative barriers to implementation and diffusion of innovative approaches to mental health care in the United Kingdom

Sir Henry Yellowlees

In this paper I start from the assumption that the 'innovations' which we are considering are those which collectively contribute to the development of a pattern of total care which will enable people suffering from mental illness to lead as normal an existence as is possible, given their particular disabilities, and which will minimize disruption of life within their community. In other words I assume that we are discussing the move towards 'Community Care' in preference to 'Institutional Care' which has been the hallmark of change as it has affected services for the mentally ill or mentally disabled in recent years. This is, of course, a grossly oversimplified statement but it is hoped that the extent to which the general concept of 'Community Care' has been publicly and professionally discussed has led to a shared appreciation of the meaning of the phrase – broad as it is – and to general agreement on the general direction in which we seek to travel.

In the United Kingdom the Social Services Committee of Parliament under the chairmanship of Mrs Renee Short completed an inquiry into Community Care with special reference to adult mentally ill and mentally handicapped people during 1984 and its report on this was published in 1985. Extensive use has been made of this report (hereinafter referred to as 'The Short Report') and of the Government's response which was published as a 'White Paper' (Cmnd 9674) in preparing this paper. Reference has also been made to a number of MIND publications, principally of 'Common Concern' (ISBN 0 90055Y 64 8) which bear on the subject.

A definition of 'community care'

The National Council for Voluntary Organizations in giving evidence to The Short Committee pointed out that the term 'Community Care' had become a slogan for pressure groups and that 'the pleasant connotation of the phrase can be misleading'. The Short Committee defined it on the basis of general principles as:

1. a preference for home life over 'institutional' care.
2. the pursuit of the ideal of normalization and integration and the avoidance so far as possible of separate provision, segregation, and restriction, (i.e. the last restrictive alternative).
3. a preference for small over large.
4. a preference for local services over distant ones.

This paper considers possible administrative barriers, under various headings, against the background of this definition.

Definition of 'administrative barriers'?

There is an element of 'administration' in any business however small and it is possible to argue that almost any act of omission or commission creates an 'administrative barrier' and can contribute to, or be directly responsible for, the failure of an organization to achieve its objectives. Alternatively, it may be held that because the acts or omissions of those who constitute 'the administration' necessarily derive from human judgements made within the constraints imposed by the structure and constitution of the administrative body, by its area of authority and by its interrelationships with other bodies true 'administrative barriers' can only be said to exist in terms of the nature of the body itself and not in relation to the actions of those who comprise it. However argument about what does or what does not constitute an administrative barrier is not profitable in relation to the problem which faces us which is simply 'Why are innovations which are widely supported and are generally agreed to be desirable not being introduced'. In examining this problem from the administrative point of view there can be no doubt that, the barriers to implementation and diffusion are – like the problem – multifactorial and will be treated as such in this paper.

Separate administrative bodies

In the United Kingdom in England, Scotland and Wales hospital services (and some personal social services) are part of the National Health Service and are administered by the Health Authorities whereas Social Services as a whole are the responsibility of local government and are administered by the Local Authority through their appointed Directors of Social Services. Responsibility for the provision of Mental Health Care is therefore similarly divided and at first glance it is tempting to suggest that the difficulties of separated and overlapping responsibilities between different authorities might best be resolved by merging Health and Social Services as a whole under one authority. However, there already exists within the United Kingdom in Northern Ireland an example of this model where the two categories of service have been run together by single Health and Social Services Boards since 1973 and, after hearing much evidence on this there, the Short Committee came to the conclusion that there were no signs that Mental Health Care had benefited to any great extent as a result of this. In any case the Short Committee believed and it would be almost universally agreed that a merger on this model would not be politically feasible in the United Kingdom as a whole. The possibility that responsibility for Mental Health Care alone might be removed both from the Health Service and the Local Authorities and be entrusted to a new unitary authority has also been considered but this would almost certainly destroy the present degree of integration of social services with other local authority services such as housing and education which is as necessary to the efficient provision of good Mental Health Care as it is to other services. Thus, although the separation of health and social services for the mentally ill is illogical and constitutes a barrier which hinders the introduction of innovations leading to the successful development of community care there is no real possibility of reorganization along the lines of a single joint organization at present. Other patterns involving special authorities, agencies, development committees, etc seem equally unrealistic and it is evident that the present priority must be to improve joint planning within the existing structural constraints.

Planning machinery – joint planning

Successful community care and in particular the process of gradually transferring those in need of care from the older more traditional care system to a newer system which receives the patient into joint care in the community is heavily dependent on co-operation and joint planning arrangements between Health and Local Authorities – planning arrangements which take account of the contributions which voluntary organizations, the consumers or customers themselves and those who care for them – the carers – can make.

There is some evidence that joint planning is facilitated when Health and Local Authority geographical boundaries are coterminous but the Short Committee came across a number of examples of good co-operation even when the added problems posed by cross-boundary responsibility were present.

Joint Care Planning Teams (JCPT) themselves vary greatly and their structures are not always constructed in a way which is likely to produce results. The Short Committee recorded one example in which it had taken 84 formal meetings, to reach the agreements necessary for a Community Mental Health Centre (CMHC) to open and inferred that the main cause of this debacle were recited in the differences in responsibility and executive power allocated to officers. Such difficulties reflect the very different structures and traditions of Health and local authorities which cannot be altered in the short or medium term. If this is so then it is of crucial importance to select the 'mix' of membership best suited to the needs of the area, reflecting an acceptable professional balance, with members of sufficient seniority to be able to commit authorities and above all consisting of persons who are fully committed to the aims and ideals being pursued. The Faculty of Community Medicine has pointed out forcibly that no amount of exhortation from central government, or pressure from parents will create commitment where none exists and an unwilling or unconvinced planner is worse than none at all.

An administrative handicap for the JCPTs is that they do not have any permanent staff and the allocation of even one officer at a reasonably senior level would make a lot of difference to the running of the teams and the ease with which conclusions are reached and decisions made. Senior staff from the authorities should always be involved.

At the level of the Joint Consultative Committees (JCC) it is again important that suitably committed people are selected for membership by the authorities.

It is also important that the voluntary bodies and the consumer voice are adequately represented and that health authority members and local authority councillors do not simply limit themselves to monitoring of financial proposals but take a wider part in the planning process itself and create and demonstrate the kind of commitment which gets results and is so urgently required. Successful joint care planning depends on a shared feeling of mutual involvement in a worthwhile cause.

Finally, Joint Care Planning Teams tend to be 'toothless' bodies whose work and recommendations are always 're-worked' by other bodies and committees higher in the organizational chain. The creation of a separate budget exclusive to joint care could have a beneficial effect on the planning process by introducing an element of greater realism. This should be attempted whatever the difficulties of joint finance.

So far as planning machinery is concerned therefore it would seem that administrative barriers to implementation exist in relation to the following.

1. absence of unitary Mental Health Care Authorities responsible for provision of care both in Hospital and in the Community.
2. absence of coterminous boundaries between Health Authorities and Local Authorities.
3. unsuitable structure and composition of Joint Care Planning Teams (JCPTs) and some Joint Consultative Committees (JCC).
4. lack of permanent staff allocated to JCPTs.
5. lack of any Joint Planning Budget.

Planning – the political diversion

Pausing after consideration of some of the barriers to progress inherent in the nature of the joint planning machinery which has had to be adopted in the absence of unitary Mental Health Care Authorities, it is necessary to consider next the effect of Politics as the administrator sees it on the provision of Mental Health Care in the United Kingdom. This volume benefits from papers on the Political and Economic Context of Mental Health Care in the United Kingdom, the United States and other countries given by distinguished contributors who are world leaders in their field. This paper in no way seeks to compete but simply records an administrative view that political uncertainty at local and national levels is seriously affecting administration and is the cause of a degree of planning 'blight' sufficient to amount to an administrative barrier to further implementation. There are 157 mental hospitals in England and Wales and a further 203 psychiatric units in general hospitals. Together they look after about 72,000 patients who occupy about one-third of all the hospital beds. General Practitioners estimate that up to 50% of all the people they see have mental rather than physical problems and the number of those in need of care who already receive it in the community as opposed to the 'institutions' far exceed those who are admitted to hospital. Around £1·5 billion is spent on the service each year and in political terms this is very big business – in votes as well as money and is also, of course, an enormous human problem.

It is all the more regrettable therefore that there appears to be an absence of political will to bring about the changes which all appear to support and a lack of clear principles on which the service should be based.

The process of running down the large mental illness hospitals has been quietly proceeding for some 25 years but it is only comparatively recently that mounting evidence that patients were being discharged from mental illness hospitals before community care services were sufficiently developed to receive them has attracted political attention. The implementation of community care policies is now a political issue in the absence of any comprehensive, clear-cut, and credible account of what those policies should be. This uncertainty is reflected at local government level where there is often a strong political element influencing appointment to Social Services Committees and Joint Consultative Committees and there is consequential administrative uncertainty leading to an absence of clearly defined planning on crucial issues.

Planning – in action

Within the Joint Care Planning Teams and at local level the absence of a clear lead is reflected in poor planning in many instances with no coherent philosophy for provision of services. Without a clear set of agreed principles the difficulties already inherent in the structure of the planning teams become exacerbated. Current planning structures in both Health and Local Authorities tend to be complex and cumbersome and it is therefore hardly surprising that planning structures between the two types of authorities compound these problems and there is a lack of effective and realistic forward planning.

Whatever may be said about the relative costs of innovative care in the community as compared with the cost of traditional care, present experience in the United Kingdom of attempts to transfer money currently expended on the *latter* to pay for the former is disappointing. Originally the concept of Joint Finance was seen as the main mechanism by which new community services could be developed and as the method by which change was brought about in services for priority groups. It has certainly had some success and has encouraged co-operation between health authorities and local authorities. However only around 5% of the total has been spent on Mental Illness, although mental handicap services have had about 33%. In recording that it was intended to develop services designed to prevent admission to hospital care, to bring people out of hospital and to support disabled or dependent people without recourse to hospital admission, the Short Committee concluded that in practice it was more likely to encourage capital or short-term revenue projects rather than the long-term expenditure on staff which is needed to support dependent people in the community. 'It has not achieved a permanent transfer of resources from the centrally funded NHS to locally financed and controlled social services' and 'responsibility was transferred but not accompanied by any long-term financial transfer'.

The practical effect of this is seen in an increasing reluctance on the part of Local Authorities to take on new commitments. However, with the promise of a major shift in the locus of care to come the giant mental illness hospitals (and mental handicap hospitals) of the past have been run down and relatively neglected in financial terms to a point at which the growing capital and revenue expense of keeping them going for longer than a very few more years is becoming prohibitive. Thus increasing numbers of people who need appropriate support from new and innovative community-based services are being discharged to communities in which neither the range, the quality or the quantity of such services are available.

The planning response in many instances has been to maintain existing traditional services for longer if at all possible and to slow up the process of discharge to the community. Recourse is then made to short-term solutions which are no substitute for properly planned approaches to care.

In the local authorities, which started with a poor reputation for the community based mental health care services – particularly residential care – priorities are determined by rate-payers' priorities and mental illness will never have a high priority. At the boundary between people who need hospital care and those who are able to cope in the community substantial costs are involved in providing domiciliary and day care services of sufficient quality to deal with the problems.

There *is* a need to invest quite heavily in community-based services *before* patients can be discharged from hospital care.

Patients and their relatives have not been blind to the lack of community-based care and complain particularly of the lack of 'respite' care and family support services. They are reluctant to have their relations discharged in these circumstances.

The general public is at best indifferent to the needs of mentally ill or handicapped people and in some communities is actively hostile towards them. The pressures on the administration can be considerable and the results in terms of the introduction of innovative community-based care, negative.

General medical practitioners caring for the families of patients discharged to the community will have a wider view of the implications of particular discharges from hospital but they are often overlooked and not involved in the planning of community provision. Sometimes they may not even be informed that a patient has been discharged yet. They become responsible for them once they re-enter the community. In such circumstances GPs may well be antipathetic to the discharge policy in general and may in any given case have a negative bias against discharge by reason of the effect it may have on the family as a whole. They can thus join the ranks of persons mentioned above whose reluctance to support the general policy of community mental health care puts pressure on the planning bodies and hinders progress.

Within the Joint Care Planning Teams therefore the absence of a clear coherent philosophy for the development of community-based mental health care and the lack of political will exacerbates the problems already inherent in the planning structure. Additional finance is not available to any great extent and faced with the run-down of the mental hospitals and discharge to the community of patients for whom adequate caring provision has not yet been made in sufficient quantity they may seek to prevent further discharge taking place where, nevertheless, community-based care has to be provided as a matter of urgency they may resort to short-term capital and revenue projects which do not meet the long-term continuing needs. Resistance to change is further supported by the attitudes of patients' relatives, general medical practitioners and the public.

Administrative barriers therefore arise in relation to:

1. absence of clear philosophy for the development of the service.
2. lack of political will.
3. relative failure of Joint Finance as a method of transferring money from Health to Local Authority provision, and lack of funds to develop community-based care.
4. indifference or hostility of doctors, patients, relatives and the general public in some areas.

Professional and other staff – the trade unions

A wide variety of staff are concerned in the provision of mental health care both in the Health Service and the community services of the local authorities. Their understanding of and their co-operation with the aims and objectives of the Authorities and the administration are essential.

It is common experience and quite understandable that during periods in which change and/or re-organization are taking place the staff of any institution or service become anxious about the future arrangements. The anxiety covers every facet of their employment and includes professional or work content, status, and inter-professional relationships as well as remuneration, working conditions, terms and conditions, and career prospects. In the process of the move from old-style institutional mental health care to community-based care, many may be asked to consider change of location and nature of work and possibly recruitment into a service provided by a different employing authority. In addition to the usual staffing problems encountered in an exercise of this kind, it has become apparent in the United Kingdom that a sizable number of staff working in the hospital service just do not believe that community care will work and assurances about job security, etc carry little weight in such circumstances.

Discussion of the roles of existing categories of staff over the years has led to the suggestion that the Mental Health Care service would benefit from the introduction of a new group or profession provided with specialist training that incorporates aspects of the training and skills of existing professional groups. The aim would be to develop a generic 'Mental Health Worker' perhaps by widening the training program which is currently provided for Community Psychiatric Nurses (CPNs). The Short report was warm in praise of the development of the CPN services as so far experienced and recommended that existing guidance on their work be reviewed. However, MIND in their publication 'Common Concern' – manifesto for a new Mental Health Service – published in 1983 had previously suggested that the new group mentioned above might 'incorporate the roles of the local authority care workers, aspects of the occupational therapists' role in day hospitals and day centres, most of the functions of the CPN, and some of the activities of the clinical psychologists and social workers'.

There is much to be said in favour of the formation of a new group of staff but of course the exact role which it would discharge is the subject of quite bitter controversy and the attitude of the existing professional bodies, staff associations and trade unions is predictably cautious where not actively hostile. The proposals for a new category of Mental Health worker illustrate very well the wide range of staff currently employed in the service and when the medical profession in terms of consultants, assistants, general medical practitioners and junior medical staff in various grades is added to those already mentioned above it will be readily seen that interstaff and interprofessional relationships are complex and can be very difficult at local level.

This paper is concerned with administrative barriers generally and it is not proposed to delve into the specific problems for individual categories of staff. Certainly 'not knowing' is one of the main difficulties and affects everyone – 'not knowing what will happen to *me*' – if it will happen, how it will happen, when it will happen, and all the consequences. Not enough has been done to bring staff into consultation at all stages. There is also a genuine anxiety about the welfare of patients for which due credit must be given.

Among the staffing problems which may become a barrier to innovation are:

1. absence of clear philosophy for the development of the service.
2. inadequate involvement of staff in consultation and the planning process, in ongoing planning and in operation and management.
3. training lacking in quantity and quality.
4. shortages – inadequate staffing levels producing stress and overwork.
5. anxieties over job security, status, job content, pay terms and conditions and over career prospects.

Planning – at local level

Something has already been said about what might be termed 'macro' planning – the planning concerned with management and large scale finance – and it is now appropriate to turn to locality planning – the planning which is about individual personal plans for people.

Here again the uncertainty about direction of change and lack of clear overall objectives has been a factor impeding progress. In some localities it had proved essential to get all the organizations concerned to announce publicly their involvement and their agreement with a published program before it started to ensure that no one single element reneged on a vital part of the plan.

Community Mental Health Centres (CMHCs) are seen increasingly as the option of choice for the redevelopment of mental health care out of the large institutions and are being established in increasing numbers in the United Kingdom. The essential characteristic of a CMHC is that it really should be *local* and should be sited in a location which the local residents themselves consider to be a focal point. Ideally, it should be close to shops and other public amenities, well served by public transport, etc. However, a new centre will often be housed in existing buildings taken over from some other function because of the high cost of purpose-built accommodation particularly at a local focal point. Such buildings are not always well suited for adaptation or located in reasonably convenient positions. Early approaches should be made to local groups and individuals who may have views on these matters and could make useful suggestions in addition to the setting up of appropriate local planning meetings of a more formal nature. No two communities are the same and plans now being made differ widely according to local circumstances. Among considerations which will affect the location of new centres is the need for the multidisciplinary teams to develop close internal working relationships, and such matters as the span of the local GP practices and the boundaries of social services' areas and other factors which could affect this, need discussion at the earliest stage. Failure to do this can produce planning solutions which do not meet the local need to the best advantage and lead to administrative difficulties which impede service development.

The concept of the CMHC as the base in the community from which care is organized and at which certain facilities such as day hospital places are available assumes the provision of mental health care by multidisciplinary teams based around community psychiatric nurses and social workers but also involving occupational therapists, psychologists and medical staff. The role of the latter has been much discussed in recent years and doctors as a group but particularly consultants working in the old-style mental hospitals have sometimes been seen as the focus of opposition to the closure of the institutions and to the introduction of innovative mental health care in the community. The rejection of any kind of 'medical model' has been a feature of the demands of some pressure groups. COHSE and NUPE, the main trade unions organizing in the psychiatric services, argue that the desire of the present government to close the mental hospitals stems from its determination to reduce markedly the amount of money currently being expended on the NHS services for mental illness by abandoning existing medical standards. They fear that big job losses would thus occur, particularly among nurses and ancillary workers, and claim that standards in the treatment and care of seriously ill patients who are still in the hospitals and will continue to require 'asylum' and inpatient treatment whatever happens require the maintenance of a variant of the existing 'medical model' with a hierarchical treatment structure and medical consultants at the top.

Whatever the outcome may be in the longer term, the controversy must not be allowed to obscure the current and continuing local need in the community to secure adequate medical involvement in the screening process as a part of the multidisciplinary approach which involves all the mental health care professions. This is a vital medical contribution and experience has shown that centres with only limited medical staff involvement are unlikely to realize their full potential.

In all these circumstances the local planning process must include scrupulous adherence to the best planning principles and, in particular, *failure to cover the following points* can and does result in the development of administrative barriers to the introduction of the new services.

1. careful 'locality' planning involving wide consultation with all concerned.
2. clear definition of the geographical area to be covered and assessment of population to be served.
3. 'education' of, and discussion with, the general public and its representatives and a positive public relations campaign.

4. publication of details of new programs with public commitment from all organizations.
5. clear formulation of objectives and policies to achieve them, including the identification of specific targets and a time scale within which they should be attained, and indicators by which progress can be evaluated.
6. clear definition of professional roles and 'boundaries' within the concept of multidisciplinary care.
7. careful and realistic costing and appropriate budgeting.
8. involvement of staff and their participation at all stages.
9. consultation with 'customers' – patients – and their relations.

Residential care – housing

Mention has been made in passing about the poor reputation of Local Authorities in general on the matter of provision of residential care for those mentally ill people who are living in the community. There are honourable exceptions among the authorities in whose areas reasonable provision has been made but where this is not the case the absence of residential care or simply the difficulty of obtaining ordinary housing is a factor which prevents implementation of the main policy and slows up discharge of mentally ill people from the hospitals. Care staff responsible for people who exist on the borderline between those who can cope in the community and those who cannot, are reluctant to expose them to the hazard of possible homelessness. Homeless mentally ill people have been called 'the invisible victims' of the shortcomings of community care as at present being implemented and this problem deserves special mention.

Money – benefits

Income support for the mentally ill living in the community, in the form of benefits paid under the Social Security Acts provisions, is an important factor in sustaining them and there is anxiety about changes to them which may make mentally ill and mentally handicapped people vulnerable. Take-up of the existing benefits by mentally ill people who are entitled to them is in any case disturbingly low and the Short report recommended that the Health Department should explore ways of increasing it. Low income is clearly related to the problems presented by homelessness and poor housing conditions and again this matter merits special mention.

Conclusion

The Introduction to this book (Chap.1) notes 'provision of effective, reasonable-cost mental health services to all sectors of the population is one of the pressing problems facing policy planners and administrators of mental health services in advanced Industrial societies' and this is followed by the claim that many desirable innovations cost less than existing methods of care – or at least cost no more. It is, therefore, certainly frustrating that 'no country in Western Europe or North America has succeeded in implementing on a large scale the organizational and clinical innovations that research evidence suggests will work'. In attempting to seek out possible administrative barriers which may be contributing to this state of affairs it has been possible to identify some areas in which administrative changes might assist in overcoming the 'block' which clearly exists and which obstructs progress so far as the United Kingdom is concerned.

Neither administrative changes nor administrative action will be sufficient on its own in a situation which is so demonstrably multifactorial. However, much can and should be done which could produce 'movement' and there is no doubt that this will occur as a result of much endeavour and hard work by people of good will and as a result of the publication of the findings of volumes such as this one.

However, although individual innovations in methods of care once they are established and in operation may cost no more than present methods, experience suggests that the introduction of them and the *process* of transferring from one system to another *does* cost money – 'new' money – which will have to be found. Furthermore it has been apparent at every turn in examining the situation and must be recognized that there are a large number of people who just simply do not want the innovations which we are discussing to come into effect. They belong to a variety of groups whose apathy or whose passive resistance to change has produced a collective inertia that has led to the present impasse.

It must be noted that this situation has been arising in some cases out of genuine anxiety for the happiness and well-being of patients and not only in response to understandable personal fears and anxieties about possible job losses, changes in status, or loss of career opportunity.

The battle to be fought, therefore, is primarily one 'for hearts and minds' – including the paramount need to generate effective political will – so that willing co-operation may replace negative apathy and that money which has to be found – is found.

Much has been said about administrative difficulties and barriers because the identification of such has been the main object of the exercise. However, it would be misleading to end this paper on a wholly negative note and grossly unfair to large numbers of devoted caring staff. Many of these have worked long hours in poor – sometimes dreadfully poor – conditions and have succeeded in improving the quality of life for less fortunate people. We hope they will soon be joined by many others and that barriers to implementation which have been identified will yield to common endeavour and fade away.

13

Administrative obstacles to innovations in the US at the Federal Level

Gerald Klerman

From 1977–1980, during the Administration of President Jimmy Carter, I served as the Administrator of the Alcohol, Drug Abuse, and Mental Health Administration (ADAMHA). ADAMHA is the major Federal agency for research, service and training programs in mental health. It is the agency which co-ordinates and integrates the programs of three institutes – the National Institute of Mental Health (NIMH), the National Institute of Drug Abuse (NIDA), and the National Institute on Alcoholism and Alcohol Abuse (NIAAA). The three ADAMHA institutes have responsibilities in the areas of research, clinical and research training, prevention, and service delivery. ADAMHA is one of the five major agencies of the Public Health Service (PHS), which also includes the National Institutes of Health (NIH), The Centers for Disease Control (CDC), the Food and Drug Administration (FDA), and other health-related Federal programs.

In this paper, I will discuss those aspects of the Federal program which relate to mental health service programs, (Mental Health Care Delivery).

The title, 'Administrative Obstacles', would usually lead the reader to expect discussion of problems within the organization, such as personnel problems due to the rigidities of the Civil Service, the powerful effect of bureaucracy to constrain change; and the power of the established organizational hierarchies and status groups to frustrate attempts at innovation and change. The conventional view is that innovation and change represent the forces of 'good' science, rationality and progress – and that they are opposed by the inherently conservative nature of bureaucracies, entrenched organizational interests, the rigidities of civil service practices and budgetary rigidities. In addition, ever present are the restrictions on resources, particularly limited financial and budgetary allocations.

While this view of the process of innovation is partially true, in my opinion it provides only a partial understanding of the dynamics of change. My knowledge of political science and organizational sociology and economics leads me to propose that a more complex and dynamic process is involved. Therefore, before discussing the administrative forces internal to a Federal organization, I will discuss some larger political policy forces in order to provide a perspective against which the administrative obstacles are best understood.

Mental health policy and the dynamics of political change in the United States

A brief review of the history of United States mental health policy is in order. My conclusion is that United States policy towards mental health throughout its history reflects larger political forces, particularly the conflicting philosophical views of the proper role of government. American political dynamics have represented continuing tension between liberal and conservative views of government. The liberal groups have advocated an increasing role for the Federal government and expansion of the Federal role into social justice, economic regulation and the provision of health and welfare services. In contrast, conservative groups have resisted the growth of Federal power, legitimizing power at municipal, county, and state levels. Where Federal power has been applied, conservative forces have tended to limit the Federal role to defence and foreign policy and have advocated a minimalist role for the Federal government in economics, health and welfare.

In this context, liberal groups have advocated increasing involvement of the Federal government in mental health and the use of Federal power, including funding, in order to increase availability of mental health services and to reduce barriers to their access, such as racial discrimination and economic inequities.

In contrast, conservative groups have supported the provision of mental health services for the Armed Forces to enhance military preparedness. They wish to limit the role of the Federal government by directly providing mental health services or indirectly supporting financing mechanisms by either categorical or reimbursement programs. Conservative groups emphasize that mental health services are the responsibility of the states and local authorities.

Historical trends

During Colonial times, mental health services were provided by local municipalities, usually through general hospitals. In the early nineteenth century, the mental hospital movement, led by Dorothea Dix and other reformers, advocated state responsibility for the creation of public mental hospitals. This was the dominant policy from the Jacksonian era through World War II. Mental health services were state responsibilities and the mental health services provided were almost exclusively hospitalization. State hospitals rapidly increased in number and by World War I nearly every state had set up some form of department of mental health to provide for regulation, supervision and administration of the increasing number of public mental health hospitals, as well as the licensing and supervision of private asylums, sanitoria, and hospitals.

In the nineteenth century there were two brief attempts at Federal involvement in mental health services. First, in the decade before the Civil War, the national census of 1850 attempted a count of mental patients in institutions as well as in the community. This census attempt turned out to be a scientific and political disaster, since the data were inaccurate and its interpretation was heavily contaminated by the controversy over slavery. Second, after the Civil War, there was a proposal for Federal land grant support for mental health services parallel to the land grant support for higher education. This legislation, however, was vetoed by President Arthur, who reaffirmed the policy that the provision of services for psychiatric patients was the states' responsibility.

Throughout the eighteenth nineteenth and early twentieth centuries, the Federal government was involved in the provision of psychiatric services for the military. The Public Health Service was responsible for quarantine activities and for provision of health services, including psychiatric services, to merchant seamen and their dependents. St Elizabeth's hospital in Washington DC became the Federal hospital for nonmilitary beneficiaries of Federal aid and, only after World War II, did its mandate become restricted to providing mental health services to the District of Columbia. Today, St Elizabeth Hospital is, in effect, the state mental hospital for the District of Columbia, but it is operated by Federal authority.

After World War I, the Public Health Service did increase its limited mental health activities. Three areas of activity are of note: (a) Goldberger's research led to the elucidation of the aetiology and pathogenesis of pellagra. The dementia associated with pellagra was a major source of admissions to hospitals, particularly in the South. (b) The Public Heath Service was actively involved in research and public health programs related to syphilis and contributed to the understanding of CNS syphilis, which was manifested clinically as general paresis. Before the advent of penicillin, CNS syphilis had a 95% death rate within five years and accounted for about 10% of admissions to United States mental health hospitals. (c) The Public Health Service developed programs for narcotic addictions and operated two hospitals for narcotic addicts, at Fort Worth, Texas and Lexington, Kentucky. Many of the leaders of the NIMH, particularly Robert Felix, the first Director of NIMH, and Lawrence Kolb, Sr developed their clinical and administrative skills and their public health orientation working with narcotic addicts in the period between World Wars I and II.

The experience during World War II provided for major changes in the United States policy towards mental health. The public's attention was drawn to psychiatric activities of the Selected Service System as well as to neuropsychiatric sources in the military.

The Selected Service System utilized psychiatrists for screening and diagnostic procedures. Large numbers of young men were rejected from military service because of diagnoses of mental retardation, psychosis, neurosis, and personality disorder. These rejections alarmed both the public and the policy makers and contributed to a growing awareness of the need for Federal programs in mental health. In this respect, it is ironic that studies conducted after World War II questioned the wisdom of policy as well as the reliability and validity of these diagnostic practices. Most of the men who were rejected from military service could have contributed to the war effort in noncombat functions. Nevertheless, the public became aware of these high rates of rejection and was sensitized to later proposals for Federal programme.

During World War II, the armed forces, particularly the army, had extensive neuropsychiatric services for their personnel, mainly for those in combat. High rates of psychiatric casualties related to combat became topics of military and public concern. The United States army organized a special research unit which included many notable social scientists. The combination of epidemiological and social science research contributed to better understanding of the relationship between combat and other stressors and rates of psychiatric casualties. The psychiatric classification was expanded to include new categories of combat fatigue, war neuroses, and traumatic and stress reactions. The military experimented with innovations in treatment of these conditions. Considerable attention was given to the use of sodium amytal to promote abreactive reactions in techniques called 'narcoanalysis', 'narcosynthesis', and 'abreactive treatment'. These treatments produced drastic short-term results but did not reduce the long-term disability. From the military point of view, the low rate of return to combat was a disappointment.

The military experience in World War II and the social sciences research emphasized the role of stress as the precipitant of psychiatric problems. After World War II, the concept of stress was extended to civilian life and stress became a major organizing principle in psychiatric theory as well as in clinical and epidemiological research.

The initiation of the Welfare State in the United States after World War II
Major changes in United States mental health policy occurred during the 1960s with the dramatic expansion of Federal involvement in social welfare. In 1946, immediately after World War II, Congress created the National Institute of Mental Health, but restricted its mandate to programs related to research and research training.

In the 1960s, during the Kennedy and Johnson Administration, the Federal government embarked on major programs in health and welfare. Although the foundation for the social programs had been laid during the New Deal in the Roosevelt Administration with social security, it was not until the 1960s that full-scale Federal involvement in health, welfare and education occurred. Congressional legislation authorized grants-in-aid to local communities for mental health centers, alcoholism treatment centres, and programs related to narcotic and opium addiction. These innovations included important organizational features. Federal involvement would be devoted to making funds available to states and local communities, but the actual delivery of mental health care would not be under direct Federal auspices; rather, it would be under the auspices of state or local governmental bodies or under newly created nongovernmental, nonprofit community organizations.

In keeping with the political philosophy during the 'war on poverty', the attempt was made to use Federal funds to bypass existing state and local authorities and to support community groups. It was believed that state, county, municipal, and other local governmental bodies were conservative and had been unresponsive to the needs of disadvantaged groups – minorities, the poor, the elderly, women and children. Federal funds were used to create a network of new, locally based community authorities and boards. Community control became a highly controversial, but central, feature of many of these programs.

The other significant change in Federal policy was the authorization of a new role for the Federal government in reimbursement of health services. Attempts in the 1930s and 1940s to create a national health insurance program had repeatedly failed. Medicare and Medicaid were enacted after intense political controversy and debate and over the opposition of the American Medical Association. The Federal funding of reimbursement programs (Medicare and Medicaid) has increased dramatically in the 20 years since the legislation, such that Federal dollars currently account for one-quarter of all United States expenditures for health.

These innovations in the 1960s embodied the following policy principles.

1. The Federal government is not involved in the direct delivery of mental health services. The exception to this principle are services delivered through the military, the Veteran's Administration and the Indian health service.
2. Federal funding for health services in general, and mental health, alcohol and drug abuse specifically, is provided through two mechanisms: categorical programs and reimbursement.
3. Categorical programs involve the provision of grants-in-aid to states and local governmental bodies and nonprofit community groups for services targeted to specific populations, such as the elderly, children, mental health, drug abuse. Federal funds are used as leverage for change through

various regulations and requirements. In order to be eligible for these categorical program funds, the recipients must meet specified requirements as to program policy, delivery systems and service standards. These categorical program regulations, however, seldom specify detailed treatment modalities or diagnostic and assessment procedures for individual patients. An exception to this, however, has been the increasing role of the Department of Education in providing funds for special education programs coupled with increasing guidelines for diagnostic procedures and standards for children with developmental disabilities, learning difficulties, and mental retardation.

4. Reimbursement programs involve the expenditure of Federal funds through insurance mechanisms (Medicare and Medicaid). In recent years, Federal Policy has increased reliance on the reimbursement program, rather than expansion of categorical programs.

The Reagan administration policies

The Reagan Administration used the reimbursement programs as mechanisms for regulation of hospital and other clinical practices through fiscal controls and through incentives for innovations in health care delivery, such as HMOs and DRGs. The Administration's intent was to restructure the delivery system. These innovations were mainly motivated by efforts at cost containment. The rate of growth of health expenditures as a percentage of GNP exceeded that of inflation. As the percentage of GNP allocated to health passed beyond 10% in the early 1980s, vigorous efforts were initiated to control health costs through fiscal, administrative and organizational innovations.

Administrative obstacles

In the United States, major program innovations in all health systems, including the mental care delivery system, (for example, community mental health centres), require Congressional authorization as well as annual appropriations for funding. Thus, the major arena for program innovations lies in the Congressional process with its committees, hearings, debates, and lobbying.

Once a program has been authorized by the Congress and funds are appropriated, the tasks are to translate the legislation into regulation and to create the administrative procedures for managing the program. These administrative procedures are inherently conservative and resistant to change and innovation. Features well known and widely discussed in professional circles which try to maintain the *status quo* are:

1. personnel practices and civil service procedures.
2. complex and redundant procedures for supervision of expenditures, such

as funding through requisitions and/or contracts, complex accounting procedures, and myriad requirements for approval of expenditures.

3. competition and rivalry between Federal agencies and among organizational components within an agency.

4. interprofessional problems among mental health professionals, particularly the competition and rivalries between psychiatrists and psychologists.

5. The power of constituency groups, including minorities, the elderly, the poor, women, and professional societies.

6. competing professional ideologies and scientific paradigms.

The politics of mental health constituency groups
An important feature of the modern democratic political process is the power of constituency groups and the political mechanisms whereby they influence decisions at the Congressional and Executive branches of the United States government.

In the mental health field, the constituent groups include mental health professionals, psychiatrists, psychologists, social workers, nurses, marriage and family counselors, drug addiction counselors, etc. These groups compete with each other and attempt to influence Congressional and Executive branches through mechanisms of lobbying, petitioning, representation. As such, their behaviour does not differ from constituency or special interest groups in the society, such as business organizations, labour, farmers, etc.

In addition to the professional groups, the mental health field has a number of other powerful constituent groups around special interests. In recent decades powerful constituencies have developed representing the minorities, Blacks, Hispanics, American Indians. This pattern in mental health is reflective of the general increase in ethnic and racial politics, particularly since the 1960s.

There is also the increasing political power of the elderly. Interestingly, the elderly have not been very concerned with mental health categorical service programs, although they have been potent forces for increases in reimbursement benefits, including Social Security and Medicare. The elderly continue to be suspicious of mental health services because of, among other things, their fear of institutionalization and of placement in nursing homes. They have not been strong advocates for innovations in mental health care delivery for the elderly: they prefer mental health care from primary care physicians and nonpsychiatric specialists.

There are relatively few powerful advocacy mental health groups for children and adolescents. This situation contrasts with the powerful impacts of groups, such as the parents of people with mental retardation or juvenile diabetes.

Advisory groups for mental health diagnostic groups have only begun to emerge as constituencies in the mental health field. The Alzheimer's Society is a fairly new organization. The National Alliance of the Mentally Ill (NAMI) has emerged as a powerful political force at the state and federal levels, advocating for the seriously mentally ill, particularly schizophrenics. NAMI has expanded its purview to include depression and affective disorders. In this respect, the mental health field should be compared to the general health field, where constituency groups for cancer, heart disease, and arthritis, have been important forces for expansion of services for support of research and innovation in treatment.

The alcoholism field is notable for the power of its constituency groups, notably the alliance between Alcoholics Anonymous (AA) and the National Council on Alcoholism (NCA). No comparable constituency group exists for drug addicts.

One of the important lessons I painfully learned during my period in Washington was the necessity for administrators to develop skills in relating to constituency groups and to understand the politics of constituencies in American Society. An important and interesting manifestation of constituency politics is the 'iron triangle'. This term refers to the alliance among three groups; (a) a constituency group organized around professional or programmatic interests, (b) one or more members of Congress and their staff, who have identified themselves with this area of interest, and (c) governmental officials in the mental health agencies who are involved in administering these program areas.

For example, when I was Administrator of ADAMHA, I attempted to undertake changes in the process and procedures for review of research grant applications and the peer review committees. These proposals were regarded as threats to the autonomy of the Alcoholism Institute (NIAAA) and pressure was exerted through a powerful Senator, Senator Harrison Williams of New Jersey. Senator Williams was known as a recovering alcoholic and a member of AA and, in his position as Chairman of the Senate Committee on Labour and Health, was an influential Senator with regard to health legislation. Documents and memos were 'leaked' by middle level staff or NIAAA to the constituency groups, notably to NCA, and to the staff of Senator Williams. This is a common experience in Washington. There are dozens of such 'triangles' and the political dynamic is not different if the issue is mental health programs or farm subsidies or military contracts.

Competing mental health ideological and scientific paradigms
An important source of innovation to change lies in the competing ideologies among mental health professionals and the different scientific paradigms. It is widely known that there is no consensus within the mental health field as to the nature of mental health and mental illness and the relative importance of biological, developmental, social and other features in the causation of mental illness. Nor is there agreement as to the major treatments to be employed – psychopharmacological, psychotherapeutic, behavioural, etc. These differences can be understood

within the concept of ideology derived from sociology, politics, and economics, or as examples of different scientific paradigms as described by Kuhn, the eminent philosopher and historian of science.

Whichever concept is employed, ideology or paradigms, the influence of these differences is powerful. These different theoretical positions are held with intensity and emotional conviction. Mental health professionals and their allies in public organizations often react to proposals to change according to their theoretical and ideological implications. Thus, attempts at innovations and change, such as the introduction of new forms of brief psychotherapy and the expansion of psychopharmacology and behaviour therapy, have been the subjects of intense ideological conflict.

Conclusions

In conclusion, I would like to summarize two aspects of my paper: Opportunities for overcoming administrative obstacles and the important role of political participation by mental health professionals.

Overcoming administrative obstacles

Understanding of these processes at the Federal level has led to a number of mechanisms for restraining these obstacles and for overcoming them. These mechanisms include the following.

1. Separation of policy staff at the highest level from the civil service program staff.
2. Administrative reorganization, especially the creation of new agencies or organizational components.
3. Use of contracts and vendorship for the provision of services outside of existing governmental organizations.
4. New program initiatives with reallocation of existing funding, or ideally, availability of new fundings.

Political participation by mental health professionals

At the Federal level of United States government, innovations in mental health care deliveries have almost always reflected larger social and political changes regarding health and social welfare. During periods where 'liberal' groups are in power, innovation is likely to occur and increased funds likely to be made available for existing programs or for the development of new programs. This trend occurred during the Progressive era in the first decades of the twentieth century – during the Roosevelt 'New Deal' era – and in the Kennedy–Johnson Administration. In contrast, during periods of conservative power, there tends to be a reduction, if not a dismantling, of Federal programs, efforts at cost containment, and an emphasis on programs to combat mental health, drugs or alcohol problems which threaten to impair the productivity and functioning of the military and industrial sectors.

Innovations in mental health care delivery are likely to continue as new technologies, both biological and psychological, emerge. The extent to which they will be implemented depends upon the balance and interplay of the political and administrative forces described in this paper.

14

The demise of a major innovation: Carter's 1980 Community Mental Health Systems Act in Reagan's hands

Herbert Pardes

It may seem obvious that rational planning, free of political influence, for mental health programs is a possibility known only to dreamers. Marmor (Chapter 10, this Volume), articulates this well and perceptively notes the national fear of concentrated authority and disdain for civil servants as forces that contribute to the frequently irrational and protracted character of mental health policy development in the United States.

The intensity of feeling, bias, and advocacy regarding mental illness is great, such that it often evokes more interest from many than one would want and disinterest on the part of some whose interest is vital. The opportunity to be in the midst of the storm of federal processes can offer a singular perspective on the making and unmaking of mental health policy. It is this perspective that will be featured in this presentation.

There is perhaps no better example than the intense concentration on mental health in the late 1970s during the years of the Carter administration, followed by the reaction under the direction of the Reagan administration in the 1980s. They were certainly different. It may be instructive but is at the minimum interesting, for those concerned with mental health policy and programs, to review the events of that era with the focus on the protracted development and subsequent rapid dismantling of the Carter mental health services reform.

The pre-existing context

The making of policy in mental health in the United States has been consistently and dramatically influenced by the broad political and social context, as well as by influential individuals with a special focus on mental health. Early in the history of our country, mentally ill people were informally attended to by families and friends through various *ad hoc* arrangements. As towns and cities became more densely populated, the pattern of family and neighbour care for the mentally ill was replaced by the establishment of organized accommodations. Almshouses and then private asylums at first were attempts to respond.

But growing needs of the indigent along with industrialization, urbanization, and weakening of communal support systems, led to a public demand for control of the mentally ill. Owing to the long-term nature of the required care, public agencies were obliged to assume the responsibility. Mental hospitals were built in increasing numbers in the early 1800s. However, in 1854 President Franklin Pierce's veto of the '12,225,000 Acre bill,' a bill to involve the federal government in mental health care through a program of land grants for construction of state hospitals, blocked substantial federal involvement in mental health for close to 100 years.

As a result, the states assumed primary responsibility, and reform efforts were typically overwhelmed by budget limitations and also a growing impression that the mentally ill often failed to respond to the treatments then available.

As the nation's population grew in the early twentieth century, recognition developed of the national scope of the mental illness problem. In 1930 the Public Health Service authority was extended to provide medical and psychiatric care in federal penal institutions, and the federal 'Narcotics Division' was changed to the Division of Mental Health (Pardes *et al.*, 1985).

It was World War II, surprisingly, that led to one of the signal developments in the history of mental health. The large number of recruits rejected owing to psychiatric problems, and the helpfulness of psychiatric treatment for many acute reactions on the battlefield, furthered the notion that a national mental health effort was necessary. In 1946, President Truman signed a National Mental Health Act, which led to the establishment of the National Institute of Mental Health (NIMH) in 1949. This Act initiated a major federal role in mental health programs, and an institution unique throughout the world.

Repeatedly, single individuals have been associated with attitudes toward and programs of mental health care. Dorothea Lynde Dix's exposure of the overall conditions of the mentally ill in the 1840s, and Clifford Beer's initiative in developing greater citizen interest in mental health, are examples. More pertinent to our discussion was John F. Kennedy's espousal of the community mental health approach. The Community Mental Health Center Program was a central part of the system to which the Carter Commission suggested modifications.

The Community Mental Health Center approach included a goal of making mental health care available throughout the country. This was to be done by using catchment areas. These referred to the 1,500 areas throughout the country which were geographical subdivisions of the state and for which a Community Mental

Health Center was to assume responsibility. The Community Mental Health Centers were to have a specified set of required mental health services. The ultimate aim was to foster a shift of the system to more outpatient care, earlier identification and intervention, and increased accessibility. This was an attempt at modifying the pre-existing pre-eminent focus on hospital care.

The Community Mental Health Center Program launched in the early 1960s had come under question during Republican administrations of the early seventies. The Republication administrations advocated a decreased federalism and accordingly a decreased focus on mental health at the national level. The early 1970s were noted too for the stagnant level of fiscal support for research on mental illness, for an attempt by the Republican administration to eliminate the program of federal support for community mental health and for administration efforts to eliminate the national support for training of mental health clinicians. This political shift from the early 1960s to the 1970s was accompanied by increasing questions as to whether the Community Mental Health Centers were attending to the seriously mentally ill. Other pressures by advocates for the mentally ill included calls for more attention to special populations such as the seriously mentally ill, children, the elderly and minorities. Concern was also pervasive regarding the absence of focus in the national mental health mission, symbolized by NIMH's inability to delimit its area of concern. While the Community Mental Health Center Program survived the 1975 Presidential veto, it was still questioned by observers from a variety of settings.

The Carter Program

These developments set the stage for the Carter administration in early 1977. Rosalynn Carter had been active in the Mental Health Association in Georgia and had pushed for conversion to a more community-based program. A Carter colleague and psychiatrist, Peter Bourne, suggested, and the President in February 1977 established, the Presidential Commission on Mental Health. This Commission, whose honorary chairperson was Rosalynn Carter, was composed of 20 prominent individuals, both professionals and concerned citizens such as the influential Florence Mahoney (she was active in creating the National Institute on Aging), John Conger, a leader in American psychology and Julius Richmond, the Assistant Secretary of Health in the Carter administration. Hearings were held by this Commission over one year in four cities under the Chairmanship of Dr Thomas E. Bryant, a physician and lawyer. The Commission assembled 35 task panels to provide analysis and recommendations.

The tenor of the Presidential Commission on Mental Health was populist, and as a result constituents emerged in great numbers to articulate their perceptions and grievances regarding shortcomings of the system. The State Mental Health Program Directors, who had enormous responsibility for the delivery of services, were critical of a failure by the NIMH Community Mental Health Center Program to involve the State Departments of Mental Health in a meaningful collaboration. They viewed the National Community Mental Health Center Program as an uncontrolled alien in what was otherwise a largely State-directed service system. Unions were concerned about threats to hospital workers' jobs. The children's groups were concerned about increasing services for children. The Mental Health Association wanted to maintain comprehensiveness in mental health programming while simultaneously urging a greater attention to prevention and consultation and education services. The professional associations (American Psychiatric Association, American Psychological Association, National Association of Social Work, American Nursing Association) were sensitive to the significance of any resulting changes not only to patients, but also to the professionals whom they represented.

After these extensive hearings, the Presidential Commission finally submitted its report to President Carter in April 1978. It stressed, among other things:

1. greater attention to underserved populations.
2. the need for greater support for research.
3. the need for continuing support for clinical training.
4. the need for greater flexibility in the development of services responsive to the community.
5. the need for better third party financing of mental health care.
6. increased attention to epidemiology and prevention.
7. the development of a plan for and commitment to the problems of the chronically mentally ill.
8. the use of performance contracts in order to foster the movement from state hospital to community care.
9. links between mental health and general health programs.

By this time, the Administration had assembled a team which would have various roles in implementing the recommendations of the Presidential Commission. Joseph Califano was Secretary of Health and Human Services, and Mr Califano had sought expertise in the appointments he made in the Health and Human Services Department. These included Donald Kennedy (later President of Stanford University) as Director of the FDA, and in the mental health related areas Dr Gerald Klerman, a distinguished Harvard researcher and clinician, as Head of the Alcohol Drug Abuse and Mental Health Administration. Dr Klerman in turn recruited Dr Herbert Pardes as Director of NIMH and also charged two outstanding lawyers, Mr Bruce Wolff and Ms Ellen Silverman, to help co-ordinate the implementation of the Presidential Commission on Mental Health's recommendations.

A decision was made to focus particularly on modifications of the Community Mental Health Centre Program. This meant integrating the perspectives of many constituent groups. It required attention from Health and Human Services leadership which had other critical priorities. That such attention could not be assumed was demonstrated in one response, when Secretary Califano had stated that the top priorities of the Department of Health and Human Services were cost containment, cost containment and cost containment.

A standard feature of any administration in Washington is tension between the cabinet secretaries and the administrative assistants in the White House. This was no less true in the area of mental health. In one instance a leader in the Department of Health and Human Services referred to the White House as an 'unnecessary level of bureaucracy'. This reflected an irritation on the part of the Department bureaucracy with the White House's inclination to direct or influence health care policy. Dr Thomas Bryant and Ms Kathleen Cade, assisting Mrs Carter, ably worked at carrying out the intent of the Presidential Commission on Mental Health. Secretary Califano's staff, torn by various competing priorities, worked in as collaborative a fashion as possible with the White House assistants. Illustrative of the tension between the two was the fact that at one point the only obstacle to moving the legislation forward was the task of drafting the legislation into appropriate language. The staff at the Department of Health and Human Services were responsible for this function; however, they were busy with cost containment language, and so the Presidential Commission effort in mental health services languished for want of appropriate personnel to perform this drafting function.

A government Task Force under the direction of Dr Klerman finally submitted a draft of an administration bill, which was accepted by Dr Bryant for Mrs Carter in the spring of 1979. Mrs Carter's dedication and tenacity helped push the bill and program forward at critical times. An example of this involvement was her testimony before Senator Kennedy's committee on February 6, 1979 in which she demonstrated her extensive knowledge of the mental health system and her advocacy for what was to be termed the Mental Health Systems Act. Her appearance before a Congressional Committee was the first such by a First Lady since Eleanor Roosevelt's appearance in the 1940s. Drs Henry A. Foley & Steven S. Sharfstein (1983) have elaborated the unfolding of mental health policy in this era in a splendid book entitled *Madness and Government* (from which this paper draws heavily). The Act was submitted to Congress on May 15, 1979. It was accompanied by a special message from the President on Mental Health, the first since President Kennedy's in 1963. President Carter stated, 'I am convinced that these actions and the passage of the Mental Health Systems Act will reduce the number of Americans robbed of vital and satisfying lives by mental illness. I ask the Congress to join with me in developing a new system of mental health care designed to deal more effectively with our nation's unmet mental health needs' (Foley & Sharfstein, 1983).

Congressional response

In the next 18 months the Congress deliberated over the bill. Congressional staff involved the various constituencies as well as representatives of the administration in these discussions. Controversy was rampant. Senator Edward Kennedy wanted an expansion of resources. Congressman William Dannemyer lamented the excessive spending of the federal government over its revenues. Over 20 groups testified at hearings in 1979 representing diverse positions. The National Council of Community Mental Health Centres and the National Association for State Mental Health Program Directors took substantially different positions on the degree of State control.

In the summer of 1979 the Mental Health Systems Act, despite the efforts of the First Lady, the various advocates of the Presidential Commission on Mental Health and some sympathetic members of Congress, was moving extremely slowly. At this time Secretary Califano was relieved of his position and Patricia Harris came in as the new Secretary. A new mediating group with Dr Steven Sharfstein, Director of Mental Health Services at NIMH, and Lee Dixon also at NIMH, playing key roles, worked on a compromise. In the Congressional setting Dr Stuart Shapiro with other staff in either Senator Kennedy's or Senator Schweicker's offices helped push a bill through, after countless rewrites and unending negotiating sessions. It should be noted that this was taking place in the context of an emerging struggle between Senator Kennedy and President Carter for the 1980 Democratic Presidential nomination. Probably, by virtue of both Senator Kennedy's family's association with mental retardation and mental health and his generally sympathetic response to Mrs Carter, demonstrated at the time of her superb presentation at the February 1979 hearings, no substantial antagonism was displaced to this issue from the overriding struggle between Kennedy and Carter for the Presidential nomination. A Senate bill was reported out in April 1980 which included increased services and increased resources as well as a focus on patients' rights, advocacy and new programs including services for victims of rape.

In the House there was still more controversy. Foley & Sharfstein (1983) point to the help of Congressman Maguire from New Jersey, who simultaneously sought and secured help with a distressed grant application from a failing centre in Bergen County, New Jersey and also remained a continuing force to see the Mental Health Systems Act through. Congressmen Waxman and Tim Lee Carter were particularly important in advocating the bill, and finally the House bill was released. It differed less from the administration version than the Senate's, and a compromise bill was then produced in a conference chaired by Mr Tim Lee Carter from the House of Representatives. Of interest was an amendment added to the bill for increased bonuses for government physicians. The Office of Management and Budget (OMB) made a zealous attempt to block this amendment, even suggesting a veto of the bill. The prospect of President Carter's vetoing his wife's bill was remote. In any event, Public Law 96–398 was passed on July 24, 1980 in the Senate by a vote of 93 to 3 and in the House on August 22, 1980 by a count of 277 to 15. The Conference Report was filed on September 22, 1980 and the Bill was signed in a ceremony in a Community Mental Health Center in northern Virginia by President Carter with Mrs Carter, Senator Kennedy and Eunice Shriver in attendance.

The Act sustained Community Mental Health Centre Programs, gave attention and allowed services development to priority groups, fostered links between mental and general health services and also initiated the notion of performance contracts with the States to foster the shift from state hospital care to community care. It included a section on patients' rights and also authorized some $800 million in new money over four years. The Act would have allowed new grants in the 650 mental health areas of the country that did not have federal Community Mental Health Center grant programs. It offered flexibility, it offered grant programs in prevention and it mandated an NIMH Office of Prevention. In all, ten new categorical programs would be set in motion. (Foley & Sharfstein, 1983).

The mental health community was euphoric when this piece of legislation finally passed. It was in fact the only piece of major health legislation passed during the Carter Administration.

The Reagan administration enters

One month later President Reagan was elected. As customary, a transitional Task Force debriefed NIMH leadership regarding the mental health programs and their status. In conversations with the NIMH Director, Pardes, the transition team which included David Winston and other colleagues from Senator Schweicker's office inquired about needed staff and monies for the Mental Health Systems Act. They also inquired about the adequacy of the current budget for clinical training. This general line of apparently supportive questioning was misleading; the actual policy of the Reagan administration became known several months later in February 1981. On Friday, February 13th before a three-day weekend, the OMB's revised mark (i.e. level) of the Carter budget for mental health was delivered to the NIMH leadership. As usual there was an opportunity to appeal, but it was limited. The recommendations included an interruption of all mental health grant programs in research and training for 18 months. The Reagan policy also included a block grant to states replacing the Community Mental Health Centre grant programs (and other federal services programs). This was deemed nonnegotiable, not subject to discussion. NIMH leadership was given until the next day to mount an appeal. NIMH and ADAMHA leadership collectively developed an appeal for more than $100 million. This appeal, over the course of several weeks, was successful in restoring the research and research training programs with the qualifier that 'social research' be eliminated. Clinical training grant programs were to be phased out over a period of time. The new Secretary of HHS, Richard Schweicker, who a short while before as Senator had been pushing for increased attention to the chronically mentally ill, was saying he would leave mental health policy regarding services to the states. Still, Secretary Schweicker, beset with countless numbers of challenging Reagan recommendations on all areas of the HHS program, was able to help secure substantial relief from the draconian recommendations regarding research, and research training in mental health.

These recommendations were presented to the Congress. An intense attempt was made by constituent groups to preserve as much as possible of the mental health programs so carefully crafted over the years of the Carter Presidency. The Reagan administration, however, had come into office on a platform of lowering taxes, decreasing federal control, increased state authority, decreased categorical programs and deregulation. Left to its own devices the Reagan administration might have had a block grant program to the states with no specifications that money was to be used for mental health, alcoholism and drug abuse. It was through the efforts of leaders such as Congressman Waxman that the ADAMHA block grant (a grant with monies earmarked only for alcohol, drug abuse and mental health programs) was finally chosen as a compromise. On August 12, 1981 President Reagan signed the Omnibus Budget Reconciliation Act, including the block grant for ADAMHA services. Only small pieces of the original Mental Health Systems Act were preserved including the patient's Bill of Rights, the development of a prevention centre, and the installation of a high office in NIMH for minority affairs.

This new Reagan policy direction radically diminished the federal government's involvement in the direction of mental health services programs. Federal care and support for the chronically mentally ill declined precipitously. The Reagan administration went further, challenging Social Security support for the chronically mentally ill as well as reversing HUD's efforts in the Carter administration years to develop housing possibilities for the mentally ill. Community Mental Health Centers were left in a far less fiscally sound position by virtue of the reduction in budget that accompanied the federal government's exit along with the difficulty in securing third-party payments which had become so critical to retaining fiscal stability. NIMH suggestions for including evaluation of this major change in its policy direction were rejected by the administration.

A retrospective perspective

One might argue that the Community Mental Health Program had brought some of this disaster on itself. Community Mental Health Centers had become diverted to programs promoting mental health and intervening in what many observers felt were less critical or serious problems. Self-actualization, personal awareness groups, pursuit of happiness and the treatment of the 'worried well' seemed to occupy too much of the effort and resources of some Community Mental Health Centers rather than a focus on clinical evaluation and treatment of serious and chronically mentally ill. But the Community Mental Health Centers did make mental health services more accessible throughout the country. They fostered local and state advocacy for increased mental health services. However, Congressional members and others expressed the disappointment of the public at the failure of the Community Mental Health Centers to prove a major factor in dealing more vigorously with the problems of the chronically mentally ill.

The Mental Health Systems Act was a compromise between comprehensive and categorical programs, hospitals and Community Mental Health Centers, community advocates and state authorities, labour advocates and professional associations, etc. It presented a complicated program, but one still representing an advance, and also greater fiscal support for mental health programs. While Secretary Califano eloquently stated the mission of the Health and Human Services Department as one of expressing the compassion of the American people for those in need, the Reagan administration took the stance that those needs were the business of other people. Other people might be the private sector, might be the states, but they certainly were not federal government, or voters who elected the Reagan administration. A dramatic difference between the Carter perspective and the Reagan perspective on people in need was nowhere more graphically demonstrated than in their perspectives on the mentally ill and in their specific legislative positions on programs for the mentally ill. The Reagan administration seemed to represent a general view within the country of disdain for taxation, a suspiciousness of federal bureaucrats, and a hostility toward individuals who seemed to be benefiting from and draining the public treasury.

Interestingly, President Pierce's veto expressed a position remarkably similar to the general tone of the Reagan administration policy 127 years later. He stated:

> I have been compelled ... to overcome the reluctance with which I dissent from the conclusions of the two Houses of Congress ...

> [I]f Congress have power to make provision for the indigent insane ... the whole field of public beneficence is thrown open to the care and culture of the Federal Government ...

> I readily ... acknowledge the duty incumbent on us all ... to provide for those who, in the mysterious order of Providence, are subject to want and to disease of body or mind, but I cannot find any authority in the Constitution that makes the Federal Government the great almoner of public charity throughout the United States. To do so would, in my judgment, be contrary to the letter and spirit of the Constitution ... [and] be prejudicial rather than beneficial to the noble offices of charity.[1]

While influential, however, this type of broad political stance is not the only major influence on the evolution of mental health policy. Some of the problems of mental health programs result from overpromise of programs at the time of their

inception. In past years, psychoanalysis, psychopharmacology, deinstitutionalization, Community Mental Health Centers, and prevention had all in turn been
hailed as cure-alls to the problems of the mental health system. This tendency is
the result of a dilemma for the mental health advocacy leadership. It is difficult to
secure attention of the uninvolved policy-maker if one does not present a policy
with enthusiasm. On the other hand, excessive enthusiasm with no detailing of the
complexities and also the potential negative aspects of such policies result in a
long-term loss of credibility for mental health policy-makers.

The Community Mental Health Center movement accomplished many things,
including a reaffirmation of the realization that people do not have to stay in the
hospital forever, an implementation of the principle that mental health services
should be available to all citizens, and the placement of appropriate services
in central locations indicating that such facilities were not programs to be
delivered and handled in isolated settings out of the public eye. However, the
notion that they would be cure-alls for the enormous problem of the chronically
mentally ill in the United States was an exaggerated promise which ultimately
contributed to public dissatisfaction with the Community Mental Health movement
and the jettisoning of the Mental Health Systems Act.

What does it all mean?

A summary of this period might suggest that a long process designed to develop
a new policy for mental health services over a four-year period was abandoned
within a few months of a new political administration. Many resources, including
time, staff, work, money, etc. might seem to have been wasted. The dominant role
of Mrs Carter, on the one hand, in the mental health policy of the late 1970s and
of President Reagan and his perspectives on the mental health policy of the 1980s
on the other suggest the dramatic influence of individuals. To some extent,
however, they also represented the country's attitudes during those years.

A caution is appropriate. Despite the abandonment of the Mental Health
Systems Act, many results that can be tracked back to the Presidential Commission
on Mental Health can be seen in the mental health system. These include:

1. increased support for mental health research.
2. an increased focus on epidemiology.
3. a central program on prevention in the NIMH.
4. a more specific targeting of goals for the national program of clinical
   training which still survives.
5. a greater coming together of the various advocacy groups in mental
   health.
6. an enormous surge of interest on the part of citizen groups in advocating
   for programs for the mentally ill.
7. increased thinking about mental health in terms of general health.

Recommendations for the future

In order to ensure support of mental health programs and greater attentions to the plight of the mentally ill, there are certain general recommendations that might apply despite the chaotic and frequently politically constrained (Marmor's Chapter 10, p. 137) position in which mental health policy-makers and planners find themselves. First is the need for greater advocacy for people with major mental illness. This need seems to be receiving more and more attention as demonstrated by the increasing numbers of advocacy groups (National Alliance for the Mentally Ill, Mental Health Association, National Depressive and Manic Depressive Association, American Mental Health Fund, National Alliance for Research on Schizophrenia and Depression (NARSAD), etc), and the dramatic increase in their memberships. Second, the mental health system should do more to present its programs based on solid data and with regular evaluation programs to assess their effectiveness. Third, it is necessary that mental health policy-makers and their collegial advocates not engage in undue optimism about community mental health care or even the current excitement in neuroscience and both real and potential biological advances in the delivery of mental health care. Fourth, it is apparent that the needs of the mentally ill vary from time to time and from patient to patient. An appropriate system of care will recognize these differences among patients and their changing needs. Such a system should be as integrated as possible, but also differentiated to recognize and respond to the diversity of patients' needs.

When one considers advising politically regarding advocacy and support for mental health programs, humility is appropriate. The political process is so unpredictable and involves so many social and political forces that a given policy-maker is typically greatly constrained in his or her potential impact. This is beautifully articulated in the Marmor Chapter as he demonstrates how the American system of public policy development is influenced by the requirement for checks and balances and the involvement of the multiple constituency groups in the United States. What is ultimately needed is a coalition of the various mental health groups arguing for the same general principles and simultaneously approaching all levels of government. This means state and local as well as federal, both at the administrative and congressional levels. The likelihood is that it will take a tenacious and powerful leader, perhaps at the level of President or Secretary of Health and Human Services, working collaboratively with key congressional members to carve out a new policy for mental health care in the United States. Some might view this as remote. However, there are many reasons to argue optimism.

The mental health system is increasingly the beneficiary of advances from research of a variety of sorts. These include advances in epidemiology, therapeutics, diagnosis, brain sciences, and the interaction between biology and behaviour. New knowledge from genetics and brain imaging, along with demonstrations of growing numbers of psychopharmacological and psychotherapeutic interventions which help are winning mental health care increasing respectability. This goes hand in hand with the increasing numbers and influence of citizen groups and the simultaneous emergence of prominent people who associate themselves with the mental health movement.

In the 1980s, repeatedly, Lasker Awards and Nobel Prizes have been given to such developments as the introduction of lithium, the demonstration of differential functioning between the left and right hemispheres, the utilization of PET scanners and MRIs for brain evaluations, the understanding of the basic biology of learning and memory, etc. In short, a more respected system of clinical care associated with widespread advocacy should help develop more consistent positions among political leaders. This has already had its effect in a steady increase in the NIMH research budget which declined by $5 million from 1969 to 1976 but increased by $176 million over the next 12 years (1977–1988). This is further symbolized by the rapid evolution of the National Alliance for Research on Schizophrenia and Depression which has already raised almost $4 million for private research efforts for the mentally ill.

The next decade will be tight by virtue of deficits and concerns about the national and international economy. However, it seems hard to imagine a more conservative policy than the intense Reagan anti-Federal position. A post-Reagan administration will likely have to re-examine national mental health policies again, and this will be done against the backdrop of a stronger system and much greater citizen advocacy particularly for the seriously mentally ill. It may be wishful thinking, but it is possible that, with these additional variables, improved mental health policies attentive to the needs of the mentally ill may be in view.

Notes

1. President Franklin Pierce: Veto of Indigent Insane Bill, Washington, DC, 1854. *Madness and Government*, 1983 p. 2.

References

Foley, H. A. & Sharfstein, S. S. (1983). *Madness and Government*. Who cares for the mentally ill? American Psychiatric Press, Inc. Washington, DC.

Pardes, H., Sirovatka, P. & Pincus, H. A. (1985). Federal and state roles in mental health. Chapter 4, p. 1–18 in Michels, R., Cavenar, J. D. & Cooper, A. M. (eds.) *Psychiatry*. Vol. 3, Section 1, J. B. Lippincott Company, Philadelphia.

Section F: Economic and professional

Editors' commentary
Economic issues often dominate discussions among those trying to improve mental health services. Knapp (Chap. 15) deals with some of these in the United Kingdom, and Rubin (Chap. 16) in the United States. Economics concerns not merely economy (the saving of money), but also effectiveness (the achievement of particular objectives), efficiency (the maximum effectiveness for a given cost or the minimum cost for a given effectiveness), and equity (fairness of justice). When we say a given approach is cost-effective the question arises 'Cost-effective for whom?'. We have already met this issue earlier in this volume. Reducing costs for A may be shifting the burden on to B–Z, which is fine for A but not for B–Z, so a broad view is essential to grasp the whole picture.

Average cost is not the only question. There is considerable variation around the mean, and sophisticated research needs to identify the sources of such variation. Community care may be cheaper and more effective for some types of problems and circumstances and not for others, and those have to be specified in detail if the best value for money is to obtained.

Knapp and Rubin largely deal with community care for psychotic patients. There are many other economic issues which we have no space to discuss. In the United States, private insurance payments account for a big slice of mental health care budgets. The rules of such insurance reimbursement crucially shape patterns of practice. Often payments are given more readily for inpatient than outpatient care, for acute than chronic services. Preventive work is not usually paid. Brief phone calls may not be reimbursed even if they avert longer more costly visits to the clinician. Identical procedures may be reimbursable if they have been performed by a doctor but not by a nurse or psychologist, even though doctors cost more by virtue of their longer training and higher earning power.

Surprisingly little attention is devoted to the all-important question of how such reimbursement rules are set and by whom they are set. Better mechanisms are needed to amend those rules to reduce costs while preserving clinical standards and to take account of improvements in clinical practice. At present, the efficacy of a procedure is not critical to whether it is reimbursed or not. Ineffective approaches are often rewarded while effective ones are not.

Drug-licensing rules are relevant. The approval of drugs by the Federal Drug Administration (FDA) in the United States and the Committee on Safety in Medicine (CSM) in the United Kingdom rests on considerations of short-term efficacy even when the drugs are required for chronic conditions over many years at great cost. It would be unrealistic to expect pharmaceutical companies to show much interest in long-term efficacy until the FDA and CSM sharpen incentives to do so. It would be a wonderful incentive if the licensing rules required that the prescription of any drug for longer than a few weeks depended on a demonstration of its long-term efficacy.

The greater costs of mental health care involve the salaries of the care providers. The longer their training, the higher their training cost and, in general, their pay after training. The latter factor strongly encourages professionals to prolong their training even if this may not greatly enhance their effectiveness as care providers. Training is then for status as much as for performance, which creates a mismatch between training and tasks performed after training. It costs far more to train a psychiatrist than a psychiatric nurse. Is the former that much more effective? What are the optimum professional mixes in mental health care teams for various client groups?

More energy is being put into improving the cost-efficiency of mental health care by delegating tasks where possible to providers with briefer training who can do the job just as well. Evidence that this can work in primary care was reviewed earlier by Paykel. The issue is, of course, not simple. Cost is not the only factor. There are complex tradeoffs in the debate on education versus training. For research and policy making longer education and status is required beyond considerations of clinical efficacy. Trainees are more attracted to a profession of higher status. Burn-out is less likely when work is more sophisticated. But the question needs to be put – what are the skills unique to each professional group, what are the redundancies and deficiencies in its training, and what would be the most economic way to assign the various types of caring tasks among the different provider groups?

Last but not least we come to a potent set of barriers to innovation reminding us of Bernard Shaw's quip that 'every profession is a conspiracy against the laity'. These professional obstacles arise from mental health care providers themselves.

Cooper (Chap. 17) divides these into those among the various professions as a whole and working within a multidisciplinary team, and those within various subgroups within given professions. Professional obstacles to the running down of mental hospitals and developing community care instead have come from medical and nursing staff, and from the organization of the mental hospitals being run down. There are many problems in multidisciplinary teams concerning authority, training and responsibility, and differing approaches to care.

To overcome such barriers, joint planning across professions has been recommended but has not been terribly successful. Cooper suggests that each discipline should teach the students of other disciplines about its own subject, and that at multidisciplinary meetings each discipline should spend some time explaining precisely what they think they can contribute particularly well.

In her comment on Cooper's chapter Test points to another professional barrier – the difficulty in recruiting health care providers for severe chronic mental illness and to the need to increase their status and income.

15

Economic barriers to innovation in mental health care: community care in the United Kingdom

Martin Knapp

Community care is a matter of marshalling resources, sharing responsibilities and combining skills to achieve good quality modern services to meet the actual needs of real people, in ways those people find acceptable and in places which encourage rather than prevent normal living.... This requires the better use of that proportion of...resources which is now locked up in the hospitals. A good quality community-orientated service may well be more expensive than a poor quality institutional one.   The aim is not to save money: but to use it responsibly
(Cmnd 9674, 1985, pp. 1–2).

Two of the most popular slogans and most important themes in British health and welfare services in the 1980s are *efficiency* and *community care*. No self-respecting policy-maker could deliver a speech which failed to employ both slogans and few published policy documents of recent years have failed to make recommendations for their promotion. To many people the two are highly correlated: a community care policy is *assumed* to be an efficient one. This assumption is as prevalent in discussions of mental health care as anywhere else. Indeed, as other papers in this volume describe, the planned run-down of the psychiatric hospitals, in many cases to eventual closure, is assumed to be such a transparently cost-effective policy that it warrants little, if any, empirical verification. And even if the assumption is correct – that is, if it *is* the case that hospital provision is less cost-effective than nonhospital provision – there has until recently been only the smallest amount of attention paid to the creation of the right policy incentives to achieve cost-effective practices.

In the fiscal austerity of the 1980s it is not surprising, of course, that hard-pressed health and welfare agencies should have looked to use money 'responsibly'. Economic considerations have been important stimuli to the search for innovatory mental health care systems. At the same time, economic considerations have erected some quite formidable barriers to the implementation of such innovations. Economic disincentives to good practice abound. It is not without some foundation that economics has been labelled the 'dismal science'. The objective of this paper, then, is to examine the economic barriers to the achievement of high quality cost-effective community care in the United Kingdom.

The public policy context

The fiscal crises prompted by the 1974 oil price saga have wrought major changes in the structure of public service delivery in the United Kingdom. The 'new managerialist' approach to health and welfare delivery is in the ascendant. New terms have entered the lexicon of health and welfare professionals, terms like performance indicators, efficiency, Rayner scrutinies, Griffiths' managers, value-for-money audits, joint planning and the like. In 1981 Her Majesty's Treasury introduced its financial management initiative which actively demanded the pursuit of the now famous three Es – economy, effectiveness and efficiency. The central tenets of this initiative have gradually filtered their way through to all levels within public sector organizations, encouraged by the establishment of new managerial tools and new quasigovernmental agencies like the Audit Commission. At the end of 1986, the Audit Commission published its detailed controversial and critical report, *Making a Reality of Community Care*. The Government's response was to commission a special review of community care from Sir Roy Griffiths, who reported in March 1988. Official comment on Griffiths' far-reaching recommendations only appeared in July 1989.

Of course, the notion of community care is not new. In the late 1950s it was recognized that many of the existing hospital buildings were old and in need of repair or replacement. Maintenance and running costs were high, yet new hospitals would be even more expensive to establish. Admission and discharge trends in the late 1950s, if they continued, would mean a fall in the number of occupied beds. In 1961 the Minister of Health issued a circular to regional hospital boards 'to ensure that no more money than is necessary is spent in the up-grading or reconditioning of mental hospitals which in ten to fifteen years are not going to be required. ... For the large, isolated and unsatisfactory buildings, closure will always be the right answer'. It was argued for many years thereafter that community provision was cheap, and certainly cheaper, than hospital. *Better Service for the Mentally Ill* (Cmnd 6233, 1975) was one of the most important policy statements of the postwar period. It included the assumption that a community psychiatric service would be no more expensive, and probably cheaper, than the hospital provision it replaced. Later, the Department of Health and Social Security

(DHSS) offered a more considered view: 'for some people community-based packages of care may not always be a less expensive or more effective alternative to residential or hospital provision' (DHSS), 1981a, p.20). Resource scarcity – perhaps more obvious today than, say, in the growth years of the 1970s, but *always* a constraint – emphasized the need for cost-conscious policy-making.

In none of the recent government policy documents or discussion is it envisaged that there will be *complete* run-down of hospital provision for people with a mental illness. There will always remain a need for some hospital places for short-term and long-term care, although preferably not in the old, remote asylums, and with the emphasis on therapy rather than custody. (Psychiatric wards or wings in district general hospitals and the hospital-hostel model arguably preserve an institutional mode of provision for and appear, *in principle*, to be inappropriate places of accommodation for many people.) Hospital closures, the Government argues, are really secondary to the development of community services. This view was expressed a few years ago by Lord Glenarthur, then Under-Secretary of State.

> Community care policies are designed to provide a better quality of life for the consumers. The Government is not looking to save money through these policies, but to use money more efficiently to achieve that aim; in commercial jargon, the customer comes first. Community care means building up alternatives to care in the long-stay hospital, providing care for people already in the community and preventing unnecessary admission to hospital. It is the creation of alternatives which will make hospital closures possible (Glenarthur, 1986, pp. 1–2).

These are laudable policy recommendations. However, the emphasis on efficiency has created certain difficulties. In recent times it may have propelled de-hospitalization forward at a rate faster than even the most committed of professionals or policy-makers would have expected or desired, and there are fears that it may be faster in some areas of the country than the speed of adaptation and response by health and social care agencies. Criticisms that policies are preceding rather than following evaluation have some foundation (see House of Commons Social Services Committee, 1985; Wilkinson and Freeman 1986; Cooper, chapter 17 this volume). Yet, the active decanting trend is likely to be more pronounced in the next few years.

The encouragement of community care, then, is based on three premises: ideologies, such as normalization; relative cost; and effectiveness, incorporating the preferences and well-being of mentally ill persons and their relatives. But it is not enough simply to *assume* the achievement of these desiderata. Policy and planning questions must ask how resources can be allocated – both within and between hospital settings – so as to achieve cost-effectiveness objectives as well as equity objectives couched in terms of normalization and acceptance. The problem is that comprehensive evaluative information on *who* may benefit in *what circumstances* is not sufficiently advanced as yet, whether in the United Kingdom or elsewhere.

The role of economics

The 'dismal science' of economics is the study of resource allocation under conditions of scarcity. But economics is not confined to the study of 'economy', nor is it the promotion of frugality. Economics is the study of those three Es already mentioned – economy, effectiveness and efficiency – as well as a fourth one, equity or justice. Every economy, effectiveness or efficiency suggestion should be accompanied by an equity enquiry: Who gains, who loses from a policy innovation? And every cost calculation should be partnered by an effectiveness assessment.

On its own, economics will rarely be sufficient to guide policy or practice, particularly in the tricky areas of health and welfare policy. Economics will generally only offer well-developed and respected insights when it works with or builds upon other perspectives. There are circumstances when economics and its attendant methodologies are uniquely well placed to analyse a particular health or welfare problem, but it is not the evaluation panacea for all fiscal ills. Economics has a great deal to offer on the assessment of costs, the measurement of effectiveness, and the evaluation of alternative care modes. However, although economics is not simply the study of economy, this paper will strengthen the prejudices of many non-economists by focusing almost exclusively on the question of costs. Other papers in this volume examine organizational, professional and political barriers to innovation, each of them with important 'economic' components.

Divert and decant: reducing the long-stay hospital population

Cutting the hospital population requires both *diversion* and *decanting*. Most post-war United Kingdom governments have put their minds, though not always their budgets, to devising newer and better ways of doing both. The agenda for the 1980s was set out in a handbook issued by the Department of Health and Social Security in 1981. *Care in Action* carried guidance on the future of hospitals and suggested closure plans phased over a ten year period if the hospitals could not provide a service reaching out into the community (DHSS, 1981*b*). Resources gained from closure 'should provide a source of staff, capital and revenue to support the development of the new pattern of health services' (DHSS, 1981*b* paragraph 5.9(c)). People with a psychiatric illness were one of the four priority groups identified in the document. The themes of *Care in Action* have been developed in later documents. Each regional health authority is now enjoined to offer a comprehensive range of accommodation and services, including secure units. Clear exhortation is given to develop regional strategies which include some hospital closures and the development of district psychiatric services. Psychiatric hospitals, though of a much smaller scale than at present, are expected to form a base for the new district services. These new developments should be at least partly funded from the savings accruing from the run-down of some hospitals.

Care in Action also stressed the need for collaboration between health and social services authorities. Structures for joint working between these agencies were set up in the 1970s, but had not been overwhelmingly successful. It was hoped that transferring National Health Service funds to social services departments, and occasionally to voluntary organizations, would provide a more appropriate and more cost-effective balance of care. In the early years, joint finance transfers enjoyed only limited success. Nationally, only about 5 % of joint finance money is spent on mental illness services, and about 33 % on services for people with learning difficulties (mental handicap). The financial benefits to social services departments were of limited duration and as fiscal belts tightened in the early 1980s, local authorities could see few benefits in accepting the transferred resources because of the various grant penalties hanging over the heads of profligate agencies (Wistow & Hardy, 1986). In 1983 the Government issued a circular, *Care in the Community*, which sought to overcome this disincentive. Health authorities could make annual payments to local authorities to encourage them to provide community-based services for people discharged from long-stay hospitals. The payments were to be financed from hospital savings and were to be (virtually) paid in perpetuity (DHSS, 1983).

Most regional health authorities have established a means to make annual transfer payments from the regional hospital budgets to district health authorities – or possibly to other authorities – for the care of people discharged from psychiatric hospitals. These annuities have become known as *dowries*. The precise arrangements vary from region to region. Unfortunately, the dowry arrangements harbour a number of financial and other disincentives to the run-down of the long-stay hospital population and the build-up of the necessary community service.

What, then, are the barriers to the desired changes in the balance of provision between hospital and community? These barriers are discussed under five headings: disaggregated cost-effectiveness, incomplete information, fragmentation of funding, valid comparisons and capital funding.

Disaggregated cost-effectiveness

Good community care – as many policy-makers and professionals now recognize – is not necessarily cheaper than hospital provision, although it may be more cost-effective. The problem is that such statements are too bold; they are couched in terms of the grand generalization and the often misleading average. For the purposes of policy and practice we need to ask:

For *whom* and under *what circumstances* is community care more cost-effective than hospital?

By moving away from the grand generalization and the reliance on broad averages, attention is properly focused on individuals, their needs, and consequences for their carers. Proper recognition is accorded the diversity of individual circumstances and their implications for service systems in general, and for costs and outcomes in particular. Inappropriate disincentives to innovation are avoided.

Individual level data are, however, costly to collect in terms of both research time and conceptualization. Few evaluations of psychiatric service innovations have analysed or presented their findings below the aggregate level. Conclusions to the effect that community psychiatric nurses (CPNs) are 'more cost-effective' than routine out-patient psychiatric follow-ups (Mangen, Paykel, Griffith, Burchall & Mancini, 1983), or that a psychiatric unit attached to a district general hospital is 'economically superior' to an area mental hospital for first admission for schizophrenia (Jones, Goldberg & Hughes, 1980), are certainly interesting and, as demonstrated by these well-designed studies, undoubtedly valid. But it must be recognized that the findings of these and a host of other evaluative studies would be much more useful and influential if they had been offered at the level of the individual patient. Are there, for example, patients for whom CPNs are *not* the more cost-effective option? And if so, are there (simple) procedures available to psychiatric service managers to identify these patients?

When we begin to examine the dehospitalization trends, which are likely to bring about the largest single change in psychiatric delivery location for many decades, we are going to need to be sensitive to differences in individual circumstances, community placement options, areas of the country, collaborative links between care agencies, and so on. For some people, community-based psychiatric treatment of provision will be more cost-effective than hospital, and for some it will be less. Given that a residual amount of inpatient psychiatric treatment will remain under even the most radical of extant dehospitalization plans we *need* to know for which patients in which circumstances one option is considered to be 'better' (including more cost-effective) than another.

Häfner (1987) illustrates this problem by noting that the total costs of 'complementary care' in psychiatric homes and group homes in Mannheim amount to an average of only 43% of the costs of continuous inpatient hospital care for a cohort of 145 schizophrenic patients admitted to inpatient treatment, and followed in a prospective study for months. But for eight of these 145 patients, the complementary care was *more* costly than continuous hospital treatment. Häfner therefore concluded: 'Certain patients require such intensive care that it is more economical to treat them in inpatient than extra-mural services' (1987, p. 123). In a study of the run-down of Friern and Claybury Hospitals in North London, it was found that the first year 'in the community' was 45% more expensive than inpatient hospital treatment for one member of the cohort of early leavers, even though the average for the full cohort of 24 was 132% cheaper. This is an early result from a much longer study, but it illustrates the misleading impressions that can follow from relying on averages (see Knapp, Beecham & Renshaw, 1987). Evaluation of eight pilot projects funded under the British Government's Care in the Community program found that community provision organized around case management principles was more cost-effective than hospital for the vast majority of people discharged after many years of inpatient stay, but a small percentage of people did *not* thrive in the community, requiring either re-admission or intensive and expensive community support (Knapp *et al.*, 1989).

Ideally, the evaluative evidence offered about alternative treatment modes or locations will be more than just descriptive, and will offer predictive advice: treatment option A is superior (more cost-effective or whatever) than option B for persons with characteristic X and under familial or social circumstances Y. In this way policy and practice can be guided by the predictive relationships and not hindered by reliance on average measures or associations. This seems such an obvious requirement for the presentation of evaluative results and their incorporation into policy and practice processes yet it is so rarely to be seen. Disaggregated cost-effectiveness enquiries, then, are to encouraged both to suggest caution – grand, dramatic policy shifts cannot be justified on the basis of broad research generalizations – and to offer an information base for the better matching of resources to needs. The fine-tuning (or, at least, the *finer*-tuning) of service responses to patient needs and symptoms should, in principle, circumvent the economic and professional barriers which are so easily erected on the road to policy change. Many of Griffith's (1988) recommendations are exactly in this vein. It is beyond the scope of this paper to discuss case management and individual program planning, but there are clear links between the growth of these modes of working and the need for appropriate disaggregated cost-effective techniques to match them (cf Davies & Challis, 1986; Renshaw *et al.*, 1988).

Incomplete information

As the value for money ethos has come to dominate so many macro-policy perspectives it is common to see decision-makers equating cost-effectiveness with cost, interpreting efficiency as simply economy, and praising anything which is cheap. The obverse of this, of course, is that high-quality services – where high quality means that they achieve high levels of effectiveness by comparison with their alternatives – often get denigrated as 'too expensive'. Yet a more costly option can simultaneously be more cost-effective. The quote from the British government with which this chapter opened makes this very point; good community care is quite likely to be more expensive than poor institutional provision for some people (and see Coren & McKale, 1985). This is another of those points whose simplicity borders on the trite, yet cost-led practices continue to abound and service innovators often face a tall barrier to change, in this case a barrier erected by service treasurers concerned solely with limiting expenditures to their annual budgets.

A second problem can arise with incomplete information. Most of the cost figures available to policy makers are incomplete. Inpatient treatment costs fall mainly to hospitals and the health authorities which manage them. For long-stay patients in psychiatric hospitals in England, treatment costs to agencies other than the National Health Service amount to no more than 4% of the total. In the community the picture is rather different. Even for a cohort of recent leavers from long-stay inpatient care, most of whom still return to their former hospital of residence for outpatient and day patient services, only some 30% of the aggregate costs fall to the health service (Knapp *et al.*, 1987). The other costs of community support are picked up by local authority social services, housing and education departments, voluntary organizations, social security budgets, and of course, clients (subsidized, most likely, out of social security benefits) and their informal carers. It may well transpire that these aggregate costs of community-based psychiatric services exceed the costs of the hospitals they are intended to replace. It might also be the case that, for some people, community-based services are no more effective than hospital. Under these circumstances and for these people a policy based only on costs to the health service would be inappropriately encouraging the emptying of the hospitals. Without sight of the 'hidden costs' of all care options we cannot expect policies to be taking us in the direction of a more sensible allocation of available care and treatment resources. And even if some of the hidden costs are not readily expressed in monetary magnitudes there is no reason why they should not be included in an evaluative study and taken into account in the policy process (Glass & Goldberg, 1977; Jones *et al.*, 1980).

Fragmentation of funding: cost-effectiveness for whom?
One of the reasons why there are often likely to be sizeable hidden costs is the fragmentation of funding of services for persons with a mental illness and the multiple lines of managerial responsibility. No single public agency – indeed, no single tier of government – has the power to shift the balance of provision on its own, or at least it cannot do so whilst maintaining an adequate quality of service. In the United Kingdom even when all services are offered by public sector agencies, flows of funds across agencies, together with flows of clients and responsibilities, must often be painfully negotiated to effect any satisfactory shift.

This is well illustrated by the difficulty of setting up community care services for people leaving hospital. Local authorities, facing grant penalties and bombarded with demands upon their limited budgets, will be reluctant to set up services for former health service patients without a subsidy. There are other reasons for a low degree of involvement by local authorities. On the other hand they may receive little encouragement to participate: transferred payments from health authorities are often made net of social security benefits, leaving little scope for capital development or peripatetic support; and local authorities often appear not to be involved in the *planning* of new service developments. Resettled hospital patients can stretch an already heavily demanded local authority service like day care, adult fostering or peripatetic social work support. What is more, a local authority opposed to the resettlement of psychiatric hospital patients in the first place, and with its own priorities for capital and other developments, is unlikely to give a high priority to community-based services, particularly when financial transfers look to be uncertain. Coupled with this reluctance on the local authority side is the limited degree on delegation that health authorities seem to be prepared to make. Dowry 'penalties' do not suggest overwhelming enthusiasm among health service managers for developing an enhanced social care role. On the other hand, of course, there is no guarantee that local authorities will use the reprovision money to develop services for persons with a mental illness.

Even when these difficulties are avoided, the joint finance arrangements in general, and dowry payments, in particular, harbour their own difficulties. If the financial transfer from hospital to community is based on the present average cost of running a hospital problems could arise for hospitals and their residents. The dowry transfers take from the hospital and give to the community. Yet usually it is the least dependent inpatients who move out first, and the cost of providing for them in hospital is somewhat below the hospital average. (Our recent estimates based on a very small sample of hospitals suggests that today's movers were costing between 80 and 90% of the hospital average (see Knapp *et al.*, 1989). On top of this, overhead costs are not saved until wards or perhaps whole hospitals close down. The result is a faster rate of financial transfer out of hospitals than the cost savings warrant. Hospitals can be left with insufficient resources for their most dependent patients.

The alternative, of course, is that hospitals hang on to the money (and maybe, therefore, also the patients) to the detriment of a community-oriented programme of psychiatric services. Many proposed developments in acute services – psychiatric or otherwise – can only be funded from the run-down of inpatient hospital care for chronic patients. There is a strong economic incentive to move the patients without the money, and that surely was much too common in Britain in previous decades and in other countries – notably the United States and Italy – more recently. The loss of money may not be the only disincentive, of course, for hospital staff – especially nursing staff – may see few reasons to participate in rehabilitation programs which appear to threaten their livelihood. There is a crying need for more qualified staff (both nursing and social work professionals) to develop community-based services, yet a host of minor and not-so-minor employment frictions reduce the flow of staff from hospitals. 'Sound manpower planning and effective training', argued the Audit Commission (1986), 'are essential. But unfortunately, both appear conspicuous by their absence'. Generally, it should be recognized that there are few incentives in NHS planning and resource mechanisms to encourage the transfer of resources to nonhealth service agencies. If, then, there is a desire to see more 'sharing of the care' between health and nonhealth agencies, the present financial arrangements in England are not ideal.

It was noted earlier that social security payments play a major part in the funding of community-based services. Here, too, there are some perversities. Health service inpatients are not eligible for social security benefits beyond a low rate of benefit for their personal needs. Some enterprising district health authorities set up housing associations (voluntary or nonprofit agencies) in whose properties residents may claim benefits. But a housing association may not always be able to offer the most suitable provision and, when all the costs are totted up, it may not be the most economical of arrangements. Another anomaly is that social security benefits are more generous for people in residential and nursing homes (in the private and voluntary sectors) than for those living in their own homes, and costs to certain statutory agencies are lower. The comprehensive costs of congregate living arrangements are also lower than independent living (Knapp & Beecham, 1989). So health and local authorities have a clear financial incentive not to offer care in domiciliary settings but in residential institutions. If, as many people would maintain, 'normalization' (sensibly interpreted) should be one of the objectives of provision for people with chronic mental illness, these social security incentives work in quite perverse ways. The asymmetric generosity of social security benefits encourages 'transinstitutionalization' rather than 'deinstitutionalization', and is clearly another barrier to those innovative changes which seek to promote normalization. And whilst hard-pressed health and social services agencies may welcome the 'costless' subsidies out of the 'bottomless' social security budgets of central government, social security arrangements are famously inconsistent. Problems with social security benefits, particularly for people with limited experience of dealing with bureaucracies and having few advocates, make for an extremely fragile foundation for the erection of community care policies.

Valid comparisons

Some policy statements and commentaries appear to forget that the population discharged from hospital over the past two decades in the United Kingdom is quite different from those who are now to be catered for in the community. Most hospitals have released their least dependent residents first, leaving behind a group of people who on average need greater help and support. In these circumstances, projections of the future burden of community care tend to underestimate the real cost to health and social service agencies and to society as a whole. The situation

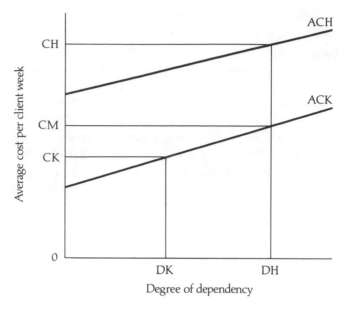

Fig. 15.1. Costs and dependency for hospital and community care.

is complicated by the dowry system. Whilst this system is an undoubted improvement on the joint finance arrangements introduced ten years ago, it has not been without its difficulties. Assumptions about any savings, including the calculation of dowries, are usually based on the average cost of hospital care, and it was noted earlier that such a baseline for the transfer will leave hospitals depleted of resources. As each successive person leaves hospital, the average hospital cost must rise, first because the overhead costs are spread between fewer individuals and, second, because the average dependency of the hospital population will rise as the most able people tend to leave first. This can be illustrated with the help of Fig. 15.1.

The two lines on the graph represent the average cost of care in hospital (ACH) and in the community (ACK). Each is drawn to represent average cost as in increasing function of dependency. It is also assumed that hospital is always more expensive than community care. (In fact, relaxing this assumption will strengthen the argument below). The 'average inpatient' is rather more dependent (DH) than the average community-based client (DK). They reflect that hospital is not only more costly than community care on a like-with-like comparison, but that the average hospital patient is also the more dependent. The health authority which seeks to resettle the 'average' hospital patient will have to find, not the amount CK, but the larger sum CM. Thus the savings to the authority of a de-hospitalization policy will be exaggerated by today's observed average costs. The outcome could well be underfunding of the new community placements of former hospital residents.

Of course, the typical dehospitalization policy not only resettles the 'easiest' patients first, but tends to move people into the community who are more dependent than the community average. The result is that average dependency and average cost go up in *both* settings. Policy-makers may thus be horrified to observe rapidly inflating costs in the hospital and in the community, especially if they originally supported a dehospitalization policy on the grounds of economy. (For example, cost per inpatient week in English nonteaching psychiatric hospitals was almost three times higher in real terms in 1984–85 than it was 20 years earlier. The real cost inflation was even as high as 32% in just the last five years. Not all of this inflation can be laid at the door of changes in patient 'dependency' – and part of the dependency change is due not to the discharge policy but to the general ageing of the hospital population – but this has undoubtedly had a marked effect). The policy of altering the balance of provision away from inpatient care *is*, in fact, economical because *total* expenditure is falling.

The alternative to this average cost inflation is that patient moves are tailored to the available budget. Only the more independent inpatients – and these are the less costly within the hospital – get to move into the community. There are clear short-term advantages in pursuing a policy of selective resettlement, but it is no solution to the longer-term problem of altering the balance of care.

Capital funding: getting started

The selective resettlement of the more independent hospital residents first has some advantages. In particular, it reduces the initial bridging costs of new community services. The problems arise later when subsequent cohorts of leavers present more behavioural problems or are more dependent on staff or informal carers for the activities of daily living, and when existing community facilities no longer have the spare capacity to accommodate them. This applies to living accommodation, day care, industrial and other 'therapeutic' workshops, family practitioner services, and so on. The marginal cost of community-based services could well be very small for the early movers from the long-stay hospitals, but the acute shortage of housing, the other demands on scarce day centre places and workshops, and the apparently higher demands of ex-hospital patients on general practitioners (Knapp *et al.*, 1987 and 1989) all combine to push up the marginal or incremental cost for subsequent leavers. Part of this rising marginal cost is obviously the capital element – the need for newly built or converted facilities, generating a need for capital funds. Unfortunately, capital funds are not easily saved out of dowry transfers (unless financial inputs from social security and other budgets allow). Many district health authorities are therefore complaining of shortages of bridging funds made available by regional health authorities. There could well be a need for a national bridging fund (cf. House of Commons Social Services Committee, 1985; Audit Commission, 1986). A further economic barrier is thus the shortage of capital funding, tied inexorably with the severe constraints imposed on local authority building by central government. It is clear from the evaluation of the Care in the Community demonstration program that pump-priming was absolutely essential for community care development (Renshaw *et al.,* 1988), yet ordinarily health and social care agencies do not have sufficient resources 'up front' to permit such an initial investment.

Leaping the barriers

One of the potentially important differences between hospital and community settings is the quality of the service offered and the resultant effectiveness of intervention. Weller (1985) and others argue that hospitals can be more effective for many of the people living in them than community services. Others argue that many people languish unnecessarily in hospitals and are ready to thrive once resettled in the community, whilst recognizing a need for the shelter of 'asylum' for a few. These arguments about relative effectiveness sometimes seem to have been submerged in national policy debates in a sea of monetary considerations. The point to remember is that a more expensive service or setting can also be more cost-effective, and a less expensive service might also be less cost-effective. Of course, we need to be aware of the expenditure difference between settings because savings from the run-down of one offer the most important source of revenue for the development of the other. It has been argued that: (a) the cost savings from running down hospitals might not be sufficient to cover the costs of setting up and running community services, and (b) even if they are, there are economic barriers in the way of change.

If we are going to leap these barriers we need both policy changes and additional evaluative data. The two, of course, are not unrelated. For example, whilst we are beginning to get a picture of the average differences in cost and effectiveness between two or more psychiatric service alternatives, we do not have very much information about those people for whom the individual difference is at odds with the average. The general point, of course, is the continuing need for empirical inputs into the decision-making system. The argument of this chapter reveals a particular need for empirical *economic* information, but it must be information which closely matches the central policy questions of the last decade of the century.

At a high level of generality these questions are not hard to identify. The policy of emptying the long-stay hospitals seems to have gathered a momentum which would take some stopping. If community services are not sufficiently resourced, and if the direst warnings of the policy's sternest critics prove to be realistic, the scandal of community 'care' may just be enough to halt it. The worst outcome would be acceptance of the 'barely tolerable' in the community. The policy poser, then, is to develop community services of a quality which far exceeds the barely tolerable but which can be financed substantially from hospital savings. Evidence is gradually accumulating to assist the policy-maker in this search (see, for example, Leff's chapter in this volume, and Knapp *et al.*, 1989), but practice may just continue to run ahead of evidence. Financial transfers from hospital to community services, and from health authorities to local authorities and voluntary organizations, clearly assist the acceptable development of community alternatives to the long-stay hospital, but as pointed out in this chapter, the present system of transfers is not without its faults. Some faults – the fragmentation of funding and responsibility and the perversity of some social security incentives are prime examples – require major policy surgery. There is no shortage of debate about such issues in the United Kingdom, and in time that debate may iterate to convergence around a widely acclaimed solution. For the moment, however, discussions of, say, lead agencies for different client groups have foundered when they reach the mentally ill, and proposals for reforming social security benefit systems for residential and nursing home care may conflict with Mrs Thatcher's government's more general desire to reduce the independent power of local authorities (DHSS, 1987). The drier of Conservative backbenchers will anyway be unsatisfied with a mode of privatization which is still predominantly dependent upon huge state subsidies out of social security budgets and will be searching for more radical solutions involving private finance and insurance and a larger role for the voluntary sector. These are just some of the fundamental policy issues which concern themselves with the economic barriers discussed in this chapter. Unfortunately, as every day passes, another cohort of long-stay psychiatric inpatients moves from hospital into the community, often with the attendant difficulties that our present administrative, professional and financial arrangements appear to bring.

Conclusion

Considerations of efficiency and developments of community care are among the most important issues in British health and social care policy in the 1980s. They are issues which come together in considering psychiatric services, and as issues they have links with the economic constraints that prompted the fiscal austerity of recent years. It is widely assumed that encouraging the development of community care is in itself a step towards a more efficient allocation of psychiatric and other resources. This assumption is confronted by examining five economic barriers to innovation in mental health care, taking as the focus of discussion the present emphasis on building up community care services and running down the long-stay hospitals. These barriers are: disaggregated cost-effectiveness, incomplete information, fragmentation of funding, valid comparisons and capital funding limitations. It is argued that these barriers either prevent dehospitalization altogether, or lead to community care arrangements which are far from satisfactory either for consumers, service agencies or the public purse. In order to leap these barriers, new empirical evaluative information would certainly help, but major public policy surgery is imperative.

References

Audit Commission (1986). *Making a Reality of Community Care*, HMSO, London.

Cmnd 6233 (1975). *Better Services for the Mentally Ill*, HMSO, London.

Cmnd 9674 (1985). *Community Care: Government Response to the Second Report from the Social Services Committee*, HMSO, London.

Coren, H. Z. & McKale, M. A. (1985), 'Community mental health unravelling: the folly of cost containment', *American Journal of Orthopsychiatry*, **55(4)**, October, 618–19.

Davies, B. P. & Challis, D. J. (1986). *Matching Resources to Needs in Community Care*, Gower, Aldershot.

Department of Health and Social Security (1981a). *Care in the Community: A Consultative Document*, HMSO, London.

Department of Health and Social Security (1981b). *Care in Action*. HMSO, London.

Department of Health and Social Security (1983). *Care in the Community*, HC(83)6 and LAC(83)5, HMSO, London.

Department of Health and Social Security (1987). *Public Support for Residential Care: Report of a Joint Central and Local Government Working Party* (Firth Report), HMSO, London.

Glass, N. J. & Goldberg, D. (1977) 'Cost–benefit analysis and the evaluation of psychiatric services', *Psychological Medicine*, **7**, 701–7.

Glenarthur, Lord (1986). Introduction and current developments. In Greg Wilkinson and Hugh Freeman (eds) *The Provision of Mental Health Services in Britain: The Way Ahead*, Gaskell, London.

Griffiths, Sir Roy (1988) *Community Care: Agenda for Action*, HMSO, London.

Häfner, H. (1987) 'Do we still need beds for psychiatric patients?', *Acta Psychiatrica Scandinavica*, **75**, 113–26.

House of Commons Select Committee on Social Services (1985). *Community Care*, HCP 13-1, Session 1984–45, HMSO, London.

Jones, R., Goldberg, D. & Hughes, B. (1980). A comparison of two different services treating schizophrenia: a cost–benefit approach, *Psychological Medicine*, **10**, 493–505.

Knapp, M. & Beecham, J. (1989). The cost effectiveness of community care for former long-stay psychiatric hospital residents, Discussion paper 628, Personal Social Services Research Unit, University of Kent at Canterbury.

Knapp, M., Beecham, J. & Renshaw, J. (1987). The cost-effectiveness of psychiatric reprovision services, Discussion Paper 533, Personal Social Services Research Unit, University of Kent at Canterbury.

Knapp, M., Cambridge, P., Darton, R., Thomason, C., Allen, C., Beecham, J. &

Leedham, I. (1989). Care in the community: final report, Discussion Paper 615, Personal Social Services Research Unit, University of Kent at Canterbury.

Mangen, S. P., Paykel, E. S., Griffiths, J. H., Burchell, A. & Mancini, P. (1983). Cost-effectiveness of community psychiatric nurse or out-patient psychiatrist care of neurotic patients, *Psychological Medicine*, **13**, 407–16.

Renshaw, J., Hampson, R., Thomason, C., Darton, R., Judge, K. & Knapp, M. (1988). *Care in the Community: the First Steps*, Gower, Aldershot.

Weller, M. P. I. (1985). 'Friern Hospital: where have all the patients gone?', *The Lancet*, **31**, 569–71.

Wilkinson, G. & Freeman, H. (eds) (1986). *The Provision of Mental Health Services in Britain: The Way Ahead*, Gaskell, London.

Wistow, G. & Hardy, B. (1986). Transferring care: can financial incentives work?. In Harrison, A. & Gretton, J. (eds) *Health Care UK 1986*, Policy Journals, London.

16

Economic barriers to implementing innovative mental health care in the United States

Jeffrey Rubin

Mental health care represents a large portion of public health expenditures. Recent data indicate that mental health organizations in the United States spent almost $14·5 billion in 1984 (Witkin *et al.*, 1987). Moreover, these figures do not include funds provided directly to the mentally ill through such programs as Social Security Disability Insurance (SSDI) and Supplemental Security Income (SSI). One estimate put the combined cost of these two programs at nearly $3 billion in 1983 (Mazade, *et al.*, 1987). Another source reported that an additional $16 billion was spent on caring for persons with mental illness in nursing homes (Committee on Government Operations, 1988).

The vast majority of mental health expenditures is for care delivered in inpatient settings. Yet professional opinion continues to emphasize the relative advantages of community treatment over various forms of institutional care. The failure of public and private funding sources to redirect sufficient funds from inpatient to community-based care is often cited as the principal shortcoming of mental health policy in the 1980s. The reasons for an inadequately funded community care system are complex. No single policy decision can be cited as the cause of the discrepancy between actual and desired patterns of resource allocation. In the literature one finds a long litany of villains and an equally long list of solutions.

In this chapter I review the principal funding sources with an eye toward explaining why any bias toward institutional-based systems of care might exist. While economic factors can certainly represent a barrier to developing more community programs, it is important to understand that program design and funding levels are the result of a process in which mental health care professionals and advocates for the mentally ill are just two of many participants. Thus, it may be more important to understand how the funding barriers have been created rather than what the barriers are. Reducing the barriers through program design changes will be the easy part of any policy reform. Achieving a sufficiently strong consensus to re-allocate funds from one source to another will be the more difficult task.

The mental health marketplace: private financing

Patterns of mental health spending are substantially influenced by rules governing which services, provided by which professionals, in which settings, are eligible for reimbursement. These rules alter the relative prices and rewards facing patients and providers. Given these incentives, patients and providers choose services which might not be consistent with current professional opinions or public policy objectives. Similar kinds of impacts are found in markets for physical health services (Manning *et al.*, 1987).

As with all items purchased in the marketplace, an individual's (or a family's) income, the relative prices for different goods and services and the person's preferences, tastes and needs will determine how much and what kinds of mental health care are purchased. For those Americans with sufficient income and other resources there is hardly any basis to expect to find economic barriers to community care. For this group, the purchase of private care, either from an individual provider or from an organized program of outpatient care offered by one of the increasing number of for-profit corporations, is feasible. The barriers that might exist for this group are more likely to arise from inadequacies on the supply side of the market.

One type of difficulty on the supply side involves the establishment of supervised housing. Creating community residences needed for independent living arrangements has proved difficult because of community opposition. In other instances, for example, rural locations, it is possible that the demand is not sufficiently large to support needed programs. The problem of inadequate local demand is found in markets for other kinds of goods and services and is certainly not unique to community mental health care. Regionalized systems of care or efforts to generate an expansion of demand are two possible solutions.

For those with low income and resources action is needed to raise effective demand. One source of funds to stimulate private demand for community care is health insurance. Private health insurance policies have placed restrictions on dollar amounts of reimbursement for mental health care (Koran & Sharfstein, 1986). Restrictions on types of services which can be reimbursed have also limited the expansion of the demand for community care. These restrictions are often based on long-held misconceptions about the relative costliness and unpredictability of mental health care (Koran & Sharfstein, 1986; Rubin, 1987).

One example of how such restrictions have affected the design and interpretation of health insurance is found in a policy covering public employees in New Jersey (Rubin, 1987). The policy provides for the extension of insurance coverage for dependents of covered employees beyond age 23 if the dependent became totally disabled as a child. Administrative officials interpreted the policy language as covering all dependents with either a physical disability or mental retardation while excluding dependents who were disabled due to mental illness. The primary rationale for this interpretation rested on expectations about the costs of covering the mentally ill dependents. Little empirical evidence existed on the actual costs associated with providing health insurance for this group. In response to litigation questioning the legality of the exclusion, a New Jersey court has ruled that, under the policy in question, the mentally ill could not be treated differently from persons with other disabling conditions.

Another approach used to increase the coverage for all mental health care has been to lobby for laws mandating specific minimum benefits for such coverage in all health insurance policies. It is unclear what impact such mandates have had on utilization of services, especially programs of community care. Typical health insurance coverage has been biased toward institutional forms of care for both physical and mental health treatments. Though mandates generally include some coverage for outpatient care, long-term, community-based care is not typically the focus of efforts to mandate coverage. A justification for this type of benefit structure is that the policies are designed to offer protection from the financial risks of needed medical care, not the range of social and counselling services usually needed in community mental health care programs.

One form of mandate which would favour community care is a requirement that a policy provide some minimum total dollar coverage with fewer restrictions on eligible providers or services. Current mandates generally require that policies provide coverage for a minimum number of visits (or a specific dollar amount) to specified providers. Often, the reason for this type of rule is that the political support for the mandate was generated by provider-oriented interest groups. As would be expected, these groups seek to limit any mandate to coverage of services they provide. A second reason for having a mandate with a provider orientation is a preference by insurers to limit potential costs and to assure that a certain standard of care is met. Also, insurers have always preferred, for obvious reasons, treatments with some limitations on periods of use, a strong likelihood of success and programs of care where there is a consensus in the medical community.

Another barrier to the expansion of insurance coverage for community mental health care originates with the demanders of health insurance coverage. Among groups of covered workers, and, in turn, their negotiators, there is a tendency to favour benefits which are more certain to be used. Recent extensions of coverage for such items as prescription drugs, eyeglasses and dental care are prime examples of this pattern. The need for mental health care, though a potentially significant financial burden, is perceived as a low probability event for most workers. Thus, there is little reward for the negotiator or union representative who wins expanded coverage of community mental health care. While a few beneficiaries will be thankful for the negotiator having had the foresight to include protection against the costs of mental health care, the vast majority of covered employees see little need for such protection.

The mental health marketplace: public financing

The private sector patterns for insurance coverage of mental health services established a standard on which the major public programs were based when they were created in the mid-1960s. Many of the design features incorporated into Medicare and Medicaid followed the then current private sector model. Fee-for-service reimbursement for physicians, cost-based reimbursement for hospital care and restrictions on mental health benefits are just some examples.

The original Medicare legislation provided coverage for hospital and physician and other services to eligible persons over age 65. In the early 1970s, coverage was expanded to include those persons below age 65 who had been recipients of Social Security Disability Insurance (SSDI) for two years (Lubitz & Pine, 1986).

Overall, a relatively small proportion of Medicare reimbursement is for psychiatric services. The percentage appears to be larger for the SSDI population than for the aged. Of the mental health benefits Medicare provides, over 80% is for inpatient care (Koran & Sharfstein, 1986).

There are a number of economic barriers to community care as a result of the Medicare benefit structure. The dollar limit of $250 per year on outpatient reimbursement effectively means that Medicare has no significant coverage for a long-term treatment program. Moreover, for the disabled, the delay in becoming eligible for Medicare further hampers efforts to enter a treatment program as quickly as possible following onset of the disability. As part of the overall market for community-based care, the relatively limited coverage for outpatient care in Medicare is certain to weaken market signals to suppliers considering establishing community programs.

In an effort to improve Medicare's role in supporting outpatient mental health care, recent legislation (PL 100–203) has increased the coverage for such care to $450 for fiscal year 1988 and to $1,100 in 1989 and beyond. The law also includes changes in provider reimbursement. Since July 1988 Medicare has provided reimbursement for the services of clinical psychologists delivered in rural health clinics and community mental health centres. From the point of view of those seeking to bring more co-ordination to mental health care this change means more of the same, at least with respect to the format for financing community mental health care. Yet, for those managing care for someone in the community, the new

Medicare policy represents an additional option which could prove helpful as part of a larger program of care.

Medicare does provide coverage for inpatient hospital care and persons in community care programs often require periods of hospitalization. One problem with Medicare's benefit design is that periodic hospitalizations could result in individuals facing the Medicare deductible ($570 in 1988) several times.[1] (This conclusion assumes the individual has neither a private policy to supplement Medicare nor Medicaid coverage.) To the extent deductibles for hospital care discourage inpatient care they serve as an incentive to find treatment in the community. But, as indicated above, the coverage or resources to finance such treatment are frequently not available.

The second major public insurance program available to finance mental health care is Medicaid. To participate in this program, which is jointly financed by state and local governments, each state must provide a specified schedule of benefits to certain low-income populations. In addition, states have the option to expand both benefits and the covered population. For mental health care states have tended to establish limits on the number of inpatient days and outpatient visits. Some states have used waivers under the Medicaid program to develop more extensive community programs.

The options available to the states in designing their Medicaid program complicate efforts to analyse the program. The difficulty in drawing generalizations about Medicaid is exemplified in a recent study (Rupp *et al.*, 1987). Researchers found substantial differences between the four major states under study. For example, the states differed in their use of eligibility criteria, mental health benefits and reimbursement methods. As a result of these differences the data showed differences in utilization, as measured by the average number of visits per user, and mental health cost per Medicaid enrollee.

The Medicaid and nonMedicaid populations which used ambulatory mental health services were relatively small (6% and 4% respectively). About 8·7% of the Medicaid population which used ambulatory mental health services were categorized as high users (25 or more visits in a year) and they incurred almost 36% of the costs. Among nonMedicaid users of ambulatory mental health services, 8·0% were high users and they incurred almost 48% of the costs. NonMedicaid users relied on a variety of other sources to finance their ambulatory mental health care. Insurance was the payment source in 23% of the cases and another 60% reported out-of-pocket payments as the source for financing their ambulatory mental health care.

As with Medicare, recent legislation affecting Medicaid will influence patterns of mental health service utilization among Medicaid eligibles. One focus of policy-makers was on correcting the perceived over-utilization of nursing homes in the

Medicaid program. The law (PL 100-203) requires states to screen nursing home patients to determine which ones need mental health care but not the intensive level of nursing care these facilities provide. Those patients not requiring nursing care will have to be placed in alternative facilities. But, as one review of this change has noted, 'Since other restrictions exclude Medicaid coverage for adults between 22–65 in facilities that specialize in the treatment of the mentally ill, this change puts a great deal of pressure on the States to increase funding for residential facilities for the mentally ill.' (Committee on Government Operations, 1988, p. 11). Whether or not this funding is forthcoming will certainly influence the effectiveness of the screening program.

The significance of these public programs can be seen through an examination of their relative importance to a wide range of mental health organizations. A survey of revenue sources as of 1983 was conducted for the following group of mental health organizations: state and county mental hospitals, private psychiatric hospitals, Veterans Administration medical centres, residential treatment centres for emotionally disturbed children, psychiatric partial care organizations, psychiatric outpatient clinics and other multiservice mental health organizations (Witkin *et al.*, 1987). These facilities reported total revenues of $11·7 billion of which 2·8% was paid by Medicare and 11·5% was paid through Medicaid. Total Medicaid spending was $1·3 billion of which 80% was paid to finance care in institutional settings. Total Medicare spending was $329 million with 90% going to inpatient care. In addition to these organizations, substantial public funding financed mental health care in nonfederal general hospitals and nursing homes.

Funding for the community-based outpatient care programs was predominantly from state mental health agency funds (some of which are federal dollars provided through a block grant) and local government funds. The reliance on the sources indicates where the growth of direct support for community-oriented programs of care has occurred. In an economic environment where public and private insurance continues to emphasize hospital-based care, the primary basis for expansion of community-based programs is likely to continue to come from direct funding by state and local governments. Thus, a primary economic barrier to instituting innovative community care programs is the limited capacity of states and localities to increase their funding support.

The ability and willingness of state and local governments to expand funding for community-based mental health care are affected by several factors. First, the states receive funding from the federal government for distribution to mental health care providers. Because these funds, provided through the Alcohol, Drug Abuse and Mental Health Block Grant, have failed to keep pace with inflation they provide little opportunity to expand existing programs or establish new ones. Second, states can look to their own revenue sources for the needed dollars to finance expansions of community care. The ability of a state to draw on this source strongly depends on the vigour of each state's economy. Expanding and growing economies generate additional tax revenues while stagnant or declining economies force states to raise tax rates or reduce spending. A third source of funds could be found if states are able to reallocate existing resources away from institutional systems of care toward community-based treatment programs (Mechanic & Aiken, 1987). Some of the problems inherent in following this strategy are discussed in detail in a later section. Suffice it to say here that, if past experience is a guide, this option is not likely to be very successful.[2]

In addition to public and private sources which directly finance care, there are a number of alternative financing mechanisms which increase the capacity of the mentally ill to live in the community. Certainly one critical element of a community care oriented system is cash benefits which can be used to meet basic living expenses. Programs such as SSDI and SSI are essential to providing the base of support to help the mentally ill meet their basic needs for food, shelter and clothing. Additional funds available to support housing programs (Boyer, 1987) and the Food Stamp program can also help make community living possible.

This brief overview of public and private sources of funding for mental health care gives just a small indication of how bewildering the array of programs can be. The difficulty of co-ordinating and organizing these many diverse programs with their varying eligibility rules and benefit structures often hinders successful community care. The co-ordination of care through the use of a case manager has been the hallmark of efforts to develop effective community care (Dill, 1987). Though some recent research may call into question the effectiveness of this approach (Franklin *et al.*, 1987), it continues to be the primary mechanism for establishing community-based mental health programs. Relying on the services of the case manager, the individual is guided through the maze of programs to assure maximum use of available benefits and receipt of needed treatment.

It is important to emphasize that trying to establish a community-based program for persons with serious mental illness does not diminish the very difficult nature of the underlying problems. Therefore, policy-makers must be cautious and be certain to institute mechanisms to evaluate the success of such programs. Even with the best of intentions to evaluate programs, problems are certain to arise.

Traditional economic measures of program evaluation such as benefit–cost analysis, are difficult to apply to programs of community mental health care (Rubin, 1984). Though a number of evaluations of various programs have been conducted, experts testifying before the Committee on Government Operations offered different views on what past research allows us to conclude with respect to alternative methods to deliver mental health care. Certainly, the extensive array of services, often required over a lengthy period of time, make community care for the seriously mentally ill expensive. Moreover, success in improving functioning and the capacity to conduct normal daily activities are difficult to value in monetary terms. Advocates, recognizing some of the limitations of economic justifications for community programs, often point to other rationales to generate support for expansions of community programs.[3]

Economic barriers to funding community-based initiatives

Whether programs of case management will be widely implemented depends first and foremost on the amount of success proponents have in obtaining the funding needed to finance these services. Early expectations for windfalls following the drastic reductions in institutional care have evaporated as state hospitals continue to receive increasing amounts of funds.

Total expenditures in state and county hospitals grew 72% between 1975 and 1983 (Witkin *et al.*, 1987). Though substantial, this growth failed to keep pace with inflation. Nonetheless, total real spending in 1983 was nearly the same as in 1969 even though average daily census in state and county mental hospitals had declined from 367,629 to 116,236. As a result of these changes, per patient spending was $4,935 in 1969 and $47,244 in 1983. Per patient annual spending in 1983 (in 1969 dollars) was $14,993 or nearly triple the amount of resources devoted to each patient in state and county mental hospitals in 1969. If real spending per patient had remained constant during this period, state and county hospitals would have required $1·8 billion or $3·7 billion less than was actually spent in 1983. Furthermore, if these funds had been allocated to community-based programs of care it would have more than doubled the actual amount spent by freestanding psychiatric clinics, freestanding partial care organizations and multiservice mental health organizations including community mental health centres.

There are many reasons for the failure of hospital funding to contract in proportion with the declining hospital population. First, state hospitals have a long history which has led to the creation of a base of continued support. Economic factors often motivate local officials and hospital employees to lobby strenuously for expansions rather than contractions of funding. It is also likely that there remains a strong undercurrent of public support for continued maintenance of public psychiatric hospitals. While professionals and political leaders speak of the importance of establishing community-based programs, public efforts to discourage local placements of group homes and related facilities speak loudly as to the public's preference for institutional care.

States were also forced to expand the level of real spending in mental hospitals because of legal victories by advocates of the mentally ill (Weiner, 1985). These cases, and the threat of additional litigation, have required states to meet higher standards of care. As a result, many state hospitals have changed from custodial to treatment facilities.

Another aspect to the inability to re-direct funds from hospitals to community care has to do with the operating structure of organizations such as mental hospitals. While we speak of the average cost of caring for one person, the reality of financing hospital care is that small reductions in the population are not likely to free up a substantial portion of operating funds. In economic terms, we would expect that the marginal cost of treating one patient is lower than the average cost of treating patients. Reducing the population by a small number does not enable administrators to achieve comparable reductions in physical space or staff. Certainly, the significance of this argument is diminished when large numbers of persons are released. When a facility can be closed or a substantial segment of a hospital can be shut down, then savings could be available.

Along with attempting to capture funds from hospitals, community programs continue to be at a disadvantage with respect to their treatment in public and private insurance programs. Continued maintenance of individuals in the community requires a stable and predictable funding source. Limits on outpatient spending in insurance programs result in diminishing the amount of available funds for long-term community treatment.

Economic factors have played a role in making housing a central problem in developing community care (Boyer, 1987). In some markets high demand has caused housing and land prices to accelerate to levels beyond the affordable range for low income persons. Moreover, recent tax law changes are expected to reduce the incentives for developers to construct and operate rental housing. As a consequence of these factors, those who are operating community programs are often required, in addition to providing mental health services, to maintain and manage housing facilities. Beyond market conditions, another factor affecting housing costs is the difficult and lengthy process often required to obtain necessary local approvals. The legal and political battles required to win approval increase costs and act as another economic barrier to community care.

Economic problems facing innovative mental health care programmes
There are now under way programs designed to test a variety of ideas as to the best way to organize and finance community-based care for the mentally ill. Whether these programs ultimately are translated into stable and continuing policies will depend not just on their success in treating and maintaining the mentally ill in the community but on their capacity to demonstrate organizational and economic feasibility.

One approach tried by the federal government is the Community Support Program. Though rather small ($15 million in 1987), this program has achieved some success in showing how local agencies can implement a comprehensive program of community mental health. Though some new funds will be available to fund additional Community Support Programs for the homeless mentally ill

(Committee on Government Operations, 1988), it is likely nonfederal sources will have to be found if such programs are to become more widespread.

Another approach has been to establish capitation programs[4]. In such a program a local agency, possibly a community mental health centre, is identified and an agreement is drafted requiring them to provide a specific set of services for each mentally ill person they agree to accept. In return for the promise to co-ordinate, and in some cases deliver, care, the agency receives a flat rate payment out of which they will fund the needed services. Obviously, one of the critical elements in the success of such a plan will be the availability of funds to enable the contracting agency to establish a capitation rate which is adequate to finance the full range of care. A solution to this dilemma would be to obtain approval from the various funding sources to pool the funds they would be expected to pay on a piecemeal basis for various services into a single fund.

The idea of pooling resources from diverse sources into a single fund was recommended most strongly in a recent article (Talbott & Sharfstein, 1986). The barriers to successfully implementing the extensive pooling suggested by these authors appear quite significant. Their proposal would necessitate the creation of a new federal entitlement program funded with resources which would otherwise go to the mentally ill through the separate programs currently in existence. This proposal rests on the premise that the principal barrier to effective community care is the organization of funding programs and the incentives they contain for selecting one type of care relative to another. If the underlying problem of creating community-based programs of care is a lack of sufficient funds currently available, then pooling funds is not likely to yield an improvement over the current situation.

Another initiative is sponsored by a private foundation, with additional support available through the use of Medicaid waivers and funds from the United States Department of Housing and Urban Development. The program is designed to aid in the creation of mental health authorities in nine United States cities (Aiken, Somers & Shore, 1986). Each mental health authority will have the power and resources needed to overcome the fragmentation of services and the barriers to community care posed by the current system of financing and organizing mental health care.

Conclusion

Overcoming the economic barriers to implementing innovative community mental health care has proven difficult, and all signs point to continued problems. Changes in Medicare rules on outpatient mental health benefits since 1988 should be of some help in overcoming existing economic barriers to community care. The increasing number of experiments with alternative arrangements to finance and deliver community care is another encouraging sign. But, even if the various experiments prove successful, however that may be defined, more fully implementing them would involve a major break with historical patterns of financing. Several factors are at work which will make the transformation of the mental health system to primarily a community-based system slow and difficult.

In a purely political sense the idea of re-structuring existing financing programs will attract an argument from those with a vested interest in current programs. Most obvious among the parties are the bureaucrats charged with administering the system and the providers who stand to lose from reforming the system. It is also fair to note that there is room for honest disagreement over the relative merits of community and inpatient programs of care.

Before any wide-scale reforms are attempted, it is essential that the results of current research be well documented. Short-term success can be misleading both in regard to program effectiveness and costs. Since many of those in the population at risk have chronic conditions, the real challenge will be to assure all concerned that community support and treatment will continue over the long term. Achieving reductions in institutional care and costs may be most easily accomplished when an experimental organization, with its own initiative and desire, operates the program. When the program becomes more broadly operational it is likely that neither the staff nor administrators will have the same skills or motivation. In the long term, these difficulties could result in higher costs and, perhaps, reduced effectiveness.

Logically, one could reasonably expect that well-run, long-term community programs could end up adding to the cost of providing mental health care. The economies which an institution captures in the areas of staffing, housing, food and other areas will be lost with community care. As many have recognized (Mechanic & Aiken, 1987), community programs cannot avoid the need to serve the same functions and meet the same responsibilities which institutions have traditionally met. Because many of the mentally ill have serious and chronic disabilities which limit the effectiveness of current treatments, community programs must be prepared to continue to provide care when cure is not feasible.

Ultimately the problems of the mentally ill can only be addressed when there are sufficient resources to fund the needed services. The ability and willingness of the public to provide the required funds will vary with a number of factors. The success of the economy as a whole plays a crucial role in the amount of funds which the tax system generates. Moreover, when the population is optimistic about their own economic future, they are more likely to support programs to help others.

When it comes to providing care for the mentally ill, there are further complications. Certainly there is a segment of the population, and it may be rather large, which would prefer to rely on institutions as the primary source of treatment for the severely mentally ill. The reality of the situation is that only a small minority of the public directly benefit from more organized and co-ordinated community care for the mentally ill. Thus, there is a need to tackle a task which could disadvantage some persons, through higher taxes, to benefit a relatively small number of people. The circumstances do not constitute a particularly attractive political situation. In a sense, even if the economic benefits and costs end up favouring community-based systems of care, the distribution of benefits and costs, with its political implications, may deter the widespread implementation of innovative community mental health care in the United States.

Notes

1 This policy was changed in 1989. Medical beneficiaries now have to pay the deductible only once a year, whatever the number of hospitalizations. Controversy over the financing of this and other Medicare reforms may lead to a repeal of the new law and a return to a per hospitalization deductible.
2 Some states, e.g. Ohio, have passed legislation aimed at such reallocation of funds. It remains to be seen whether these laws will be effective and whether other states will pass similar laws.
3 The effects of long-term institutionalization, prevention of homelessness, and wish to guarantee basic civil liberties are among the non-economic rationales for community care.
4 For a detailed description of recent efforts, see Mechanic & Aiken (1989).

Acknowledgements

The author thanks David Mechanic for helpful comments. Support from the Rutgers Center for Research on the Organization and Financing of Care for the Severely Mentally Ill, and NIMH Grant No. NH43450-01, is gratefully acknowledged.

References

Aiken, L. H., Somers, S. A. & Shore, M. F. (1986). Private Foundations in Health Affairs: A Case Study of the Development of a National Initiative for the Chronically Mentally Ill, *American Psychologist*, **41**, 1290–5.
Boyer, C. A. (1987). Obstacles in Urban Housing Policy for the Chronically Mentally Ill. In (D. Mechanic, ed.) *Improving Mental Health Services: What the Social Sciences Can Tell Us*, pp. 71–81. Jossey-Bass Inc.: San Francisco.
Committee on Government Operations (1988). From Back Wards to Back Streets: The Failure of the Federal Government in Providing Services for the Mentally Ill, House Report 100–541, US Government Printing Office, Washington, DC.
Dill, A. E. P. (1987). Issues in Case Management for the Chronically Mentally Ill. In (D. Mechanic, ed.) *Improving Mental Health Services: What the Social Sciences Can Tell Us*, pp. 61–70, Jossey-Bass Inc.: San Francisco.
Franklin, J. L., Solovitz, B., Mason, M., Clemons, J. R. & Miller, G. E. (1987). An Evaluation of Case Management, *American Journal of Public Health*, **77 (6)** 674–8.

Koran, L. M. & Sharfstein, S. S. (1986). Mental Health Services, In S. Jonas with contributors, *Health Care Delivery in the United States*, 3rd edn, pp. 263–302, Springer Publishing Company: New York.

Lubitz, J. & Pine, P. (1986). Health Care Use by Medicare's Disabled Enrollees, *Health Care Financing Review*, **7 (4)**, 19–30.

Manning, M., Newhouse, J., Duan, N., Keeler, E., Leibowitz, A. & Marquis, M. (1987). Health Insurance and the Demand for Medical Care: Evidence from a Randomized Experiment, *American Economic Review*, **77 (3)**, 251–77.

Mazade, N. A., Lutterman, T., Wurster, C. R. & Glover, R. W. (1987). State and Federal Expenditures for Mental Health Services, United States, 1983. In National Institute of Mental Health. *Mental Health, United States, 1987* (R. W. Manderscheid and S. A. Barrett, eds) DHHS Pub. No. (ADM) 87-1518, pp. 144–57. Washington, D.C.: Supt. of Docs., US Govt. Print. Off.

Mechanic, D. & Aiken, L. eds. (1989) *Paying for Services: Promises and Pitfalls of Capitation*. Jossey-Bass Inc.: San Francisco.

Mechanic, D. & Aiken, L. (1987). Improving the Care of Patients with Chronic Mental Illness, *New England Journal of Medicine*, **317**, 1634–8.

Rubin, J. (1983). Benefit–Cost Analysis and the Care of the Chronic Psychiatric Patient in the Community. In (I. Barofsky and R. Budson, eds), *The Chronic Psychiatric Patient in the Community: Principles of Treatment*, pp. 457–74. SP Medical and Scientific Books, New York.

Rubin, J. (1987). Discrimination and Insurance Coverage of the Mentally Ill. In (R. Scheffler and T. McGuire, eds), *Research Issues in Economics and Mental Health*, pp. 195–209. JAI Press, Greenwich, Conn.

Rupp. A., Taube, C. A., Bodison, D. & Barrett, S. A. (1987). Medicaid and Ambulatory Mental Health Care: Utilization and Costs. In National Institute of Mental Health. *Mental Health, United States, 1987*. (R. W. Manderscheid and S. A. Barrett, eds), pp. 187–204. DHHS Pub. No. (ADM) 87-1518. Washington, DC: Supt. of Docs., US Govt. Print. Off.

Talbott, J. A. & Sharfstein, S. (1986). A Proposal for Future Funding of Chronic and Episodic Mental Illness, *Hospital and Community Psychiatry*, **37 (11)**, 1126–30.

Weiner, B. A. (1985). Treatment Rights. In (S. J. Brakel, J. Parry and B. A. Weiner, eds), *The Mentally Disabled and the Law*, 3rd edn, pp. 327–67. American Bar Foundation: Chicago.

Witkin, M. J., Atay, J. E., Fell, A. S. & Manderscheid, R. W. (1987). Specialty Mental Health System Characteristics. In National Institute of Mental Health. *Mental Health, United States, 1987*. (R. W. Manderscheid and S. A. Barrett, eds), pp. 14–58. DHHS Pub. No. (ADM) 87–1518. Washington, DC: Supt. of Docs., US Govt. Print Off.

17

Professional obstacles to implementation and diffusion of innovative approaches to mental health care

John E. Cooper

Two quite broad and complicated issues have been selected from the numerous possibilities. The issues selected are as follows.

1.   The move of psychiatric services and patients away from large institutions, into a network of services and facilities nearer to the homes of the patients. This has conventionally been called 'Community Psychiatry', but in its more fully developed forms is perhaps better called 'Neighbourhood Psychiatry'.
2.   The development of a style of work based upon a multidisciplinary team. This raises a variety of problems to do with the separation and blurring of professional roles, the allocation of responsibility, and leadership. In some respects these two major types of development can be discussed separately but in practice they are very closely connected as the major components of a 'package deal' of a new style of community or neighbourhood psychiatry. This new style of work is associated with a complex of attitudes and practices that is typical of a new generation of psychiatrists and mental health workers.

In discussing these issues, I shall occasionally divide the discussion up into:

1. problems between the different professions (namely, psychiatry, social work, psychology, nursing and occupational therapy) in the sense of problems identified as matters of principle in the debate between representatives of the different professional organizations.
2. problems between individuals of these different professions in their daily work as members of the same multidisciplinary team.

3. problems between specialists within the medical profession, particularly between psychiatrists of different generations and between psychiatrists and general practitioners.

Experience shows that many health workers and administrators in the United States are not fully aware of some of the characteristics of the National Health Service in the United Kingdom that have an important bearing on many of the issues discussed here. Two short introductory sections have therefore been included that deal with the main clinical components of the National Health Service, and some related points about my own clinical experience working within it.

Personal viewpoint and clinical experience

I am what is known in the United Kingdom as an academic clinician. That is to say my primary responsibility is to teach undergraduate medical students a psychologically minded approach to all types of patients, plus some basic clinical psychiatry. I am also expected to do some research. Universities in the United Kingdom pay professors of clinical medical disciplines all at the same rate, which is the same as all consultant physicians in the National Health Service. To do this teaching and research it is necessary to have access to clinical facilities and patients, and this is obtained by having a roughly half-time honorary (i.e. unpaid) clinical contract within the National Health Service. This clinical work is done alongside the full-time National Health Service consultants, in the same premises and under the same conditions of work. Although professors of psychiatry in medical schools are heads of the academic departments, we have no authority at all over the clinical or research work of our NHS consultant colleagues, even those working alongside us in the specified university teaching hospitals. This is quite unlike the position in many universities in the United States and on the continent of Europe. My clinical experience that is of relevance to this discussion is a period of twelve years working entirely from a mental hospital base (Mapperley Hospital, Nottingham) and the last two years working in the acute psychiatric unit in a new University Hospital. I have never worked as a clinician in the United States but I have observed the American scene on a number of occasions and have had many discussions of these problems with American colleagues. Most of the points raised in this chapter will be found to be relevant to the American scene, and this is particularly so for those parts of the United States where various forms of prospective payment or Health Maintenance Organizations have been or are being developed. These are very patchy in their distribution and there are several varieties in existence: however, they seem to be numerous and important and may be even more so in the future. The multidisciplinary teams discussed and defined here are broadly similar to those in the Community Mental Health Centres that were so prominent in the United States some years ago, and also to the teams still found in crisis intervention units, accident and emergency departments, and rehabilitation units in both the United States and Europe.

The main clinical components of the National Health Service in the United Kingdom
The two major components of the British National Health Service are the hospital services, and the general practitioner services; these are loosely linked together under the overall National Health Service, but they operate more or less independently. The unifying principles of both these major components of the NHS are that, from the point of view of the patient, they are very largely free, they are easy of access, and they are comprehensive. The hospital consultants are paid a set salary which depends upon seniority, and all the staff of the different medical specialties are paid at the same rate. General practitioners are individually contracted to a separate Family Practitioner Committee and are paid partly on a capitation fee basis, i.e. for each patient on their list they receive a fixed annual sum. This does not vary with the number or type of services used, and so it makes no difference to the salary of a general practitioner whether he sees a patient once or 20 times in a year, or whether the patient has multiple investigations and operations or nothing at all.

Although the consultants and general practitioners have these very different arrangements, the practical result is that neither the general practitioner nor consultant has to worry on behalf of the patient about the cost of the service they are providing. Similarly, the amount of work done does not affect the salary of the doctor. This is a great advantage to the doctors and other professionals in planning treatment programs and is probably one of the main reasons why somewhat lower salaries in the United Kingdom are accepted compared to the United States although this acceptance is changing as a result of the Conservative Government's promotion of private practice over the last decade. Personally, I would find it very difficult to make decisions about how many times to see a patient and what medication or investigations to order, if I knew that this would cause severe financial problems, or would increase my own financial rewards. (I have, in fact, during my career, done two short periods of private practice while 'resting' between NHS appointments, and I found these issues to be quite difficult problems.)

In spite of the wishes and efforts of the present government, the extent of private practice in the United Kingdom is still limited. Consultants of all disciplines are now permitted to earn an amount equivalent to up to a maximum of 10% of their National Health Service salary by private practice, but it is noteworthy that the majority still do not bother to take up this option – particularly in psychiatry.

In general, the National Health Service in the United Kingdom can be seen as being designed for the benefit of the patient (it was brought into being by a labour government against the wishes of large sections of the medical profession). This contrasts with the health services in the United States which appear to be designed for the convenience and benefit of the doctors. (The health services of most of the Eastern European countries seem different again, in that they appear to be designed for the convenience of the state bureaucracy; neither the patient nor the doctor gets the best of the deal.)

The nature of and reasons for major strategic changes in the psychiatric services in the United Kingdom

For the last 20 years or more, it has been a major National, Regional and District policy within the National Health Service to attempt gradually to lessen the dependence of the psychiatric services upon the 200 or so Victorian style institutions that are scattered around the country. In 1965, it was officially announced that by 1970 some 20 specified large mental hospitals would be closed. Twenty years later, by 1986, the closure score was one, but there has been extensive decrease in the number of mental hospital inpatients and change in the nature of the services and the orientation of those working in them. A parallel policy has been to set up acute psychiatric units on district general hospital sites, although we are still a long way from replacing all the acute facilities in this way. A major point to be made here is that these two major points of strategic policy were not arrived at by means of evaluative studies, or by careful examination of the needs of the community (or even by considering the views of the psychiatrists). They were adopted simply because they seemed reasonable and attractive from several points of view, and because they have a very obviously humane feel about them. Equally the discharge of large numbers of long-stay patients from institutional care into smaller hostels, halfway houses and other facilities (including the patients' homes) was set in motion long before any evaluations were made. It is difficult to know whether these new strategies will turn out in the long run to be cheaper or more expensive than the old style of institutional care. The obvious short-term savings on building maintenance and estate costs are easily swallowed up by the need for more and better trained staff and the higher standards of living of the patients in modern units must cost more than the often minimal standards of the large hospitals. Some costs are also transferred to friends, relatives and the General Practitioner service, rather than abolished. Test (this volume) has studied some community schemes which do not work out more expensive than institutional care, but it is not necessarily legitimate to generalise from one scheme or one country to another. Much will depend upon the level of disability of the patients being moved; the first few hundred long-stay patients moved out of a large institution will be those with the less severe degrees of social and physical disabilities, and they will therefore have less expensive needs than the remainder.

The same lack of evaluation before being put into practice applies to working in multidisciplinary teams. This instance is perhaps understandable, since multidisciplinary team work can be interpreted as a more or less inevitable consequence of increasing numbers and varieties of professional staff trying to cope with patients and families outside the restrictions of an institution; there are many clear examples of this in the literature on crisis intervention (Cooper, 1979). This process continues, and in the United Kingdom at the moment there is an abundance of meetings and conferences on multidisciplinary team work and relationships between professions, usually organized by members of the social work and nursing professions as they realise they are being given more and more responsibility for more and more awkward problems.

Another important historical point is that the changes in mental hospital populations in the United Kingdom, although in the same direction as those in the United States have been occurring at a different pace. In some parts of the United States, and in Italy, there have been a number of sudden administrative or statutory changes which have produced sudden outpourings of long-stay mental hospital patients into unprepared communities. The so-called 'Italian experience' following the national legislation of 1978 is the most spectacular recent example of this. By contrast, in the United Kingdom there has been a steady decline in the long-stay populations in almost all the mental hospitals, and few sudden surges forced by unexpected administrative or legal changes. Adequate accommodation in a variety of locations in the community has usually been provided for the patients, together with varying degrees of support from developing community psychiatric nurse services; an increased input from general practitioners is also available. Rehabilitation units, sheltered industrial workshops, and a variety of day centres and day hospitals have also been developed, so that there has been relatively little vagrancy, neglect and social isolation in these discharged patients. The experience in the United Kingdom is that whatever is done for patients of this type a small number inevitably drift away from the service and turn up, sometimes years later, in a neglected and isolated state in spite of all possible efforts to keep in contact with them. These unfortunate patients are the ones that are triumphantly produced and described by journalists, television programs, and workers for MIND, who then accuse the local psychiatrists of ejecting these patients abruptly from the comfortable psychiatric hospitals. If these critics of the psychiatric services were to sit down and spend a few hours talking to these same patients, trying to persuade them to engage in ordinary everyday activities, they might begin to see some of the problems.

This fairly smooth rate of run-down of large mental hospitals in the United Kingdom is now likely to change, as the actual closure of many hospitals approaches. The administrative, financial and professional problems associated with this phase will be discussed later, but it is becoming clear that the costs and the problems associated with the closure, as opposed to the running down, are of a new order of magnitude.

Professional obstacles to the development of community care
Private practice
There are good grounds for believing that in some circumstances a dominant private care element in a health service could produce a strong block to this type of move. The reference here is to privately run small psychiatric hospitals, of the sort that are now being developed in the United Kingdom as a result of governmental pressure in favour of an increase in the private element in the National Health Service. No doubt there are a large variety of similar small private institutions in the United States, and those in Japan have recently been exposed to considerable publicity and criticism. The basic difficulty seems to be that to make a profit, a private psychiatric hospital has to remain as full as possible since an empty bed represents a loss of potential fees. In addition, the more investigations and examinations that are performed, the bigger the profit for all concerned. Avoidance of a spell in hospital by energetic crisis intervention or by domiciliary visiting is not financially attractive for staff based in the hospital.

Resistance from medical and nursing staff
Even within a National Health Service free from these financial forces, there are instances to be seen of professional obstacles to both the running down and the closure of large psychiatric institutions. Many of the present senior generation of psychiatrists in the United Kingdom have had experience of trying to change single-sex wards with locked doors, into wards with unlocked doors and with day facilities shared by the sexes. Although it is commonly found that, once these changes have been made, both the patients and the nursing staff function very much better, there is almost always a resistance to this change from the more senior members of the nursing profession, and sometimes even from the more senior psychiatrists. Once this phase has been worked through there is often another phase of more subtle difficulties when attempts are made to break down some of the more benign aspects of the institution. I am referring to the development of small groups of often quite elderly and sometimes also frail patients in 'villas' or comfortably furnished and decorated long-stay hospital wards, in which the population becomes stable, comfortable and well socialised. Far from being in frequent need of the attentions of a psychiatrist, patients of this type become puzzled and anxious (and so do the nursing staff in charge of them) if interviewed more than once every three months by their consultant. A number of patients under these conditions are often found to be valuable members of the workforce of the ward, or of domestic services in the hospital. I have had personal experience of trying to get institutionalized nursing staff to accept that most of the patients in this type of long-stay ward would be just as happy outside the hospital in a smaller, domestic style of accommodation. It usually takes somewhere between one and two years to work through and change these attitudes and to achieve significant

numbers of discharges and relocations. As already noted, success depends partly upon increased interaction with the individual patients and the nursing staff, and partly upon the provision of additional professional staff such as social workers, occupational therapists and psychologists; they are needed to share the workload and keep up the pressure that gradually breaks down the benign paralysis of the comfortable long-stay ward. An adequate long-term follow up system is also required for some of the patients once they have moved out, and a good deal of co-operation with the local Social Services (which in England are outside the National Health Service) is necessary. This whole process is, of course, in some respects no more than a transfer of the burden of care to other facilities and other services. In the United Kingdom some mental hospitals now find themselves hosts to long-stay patients suitable for transfer to smaller-scale accommodation in two or three different Health Districts. The necessary communication and co-operation between the large hospital and the several District Authorities is often slow or nonexistent, although in theory the Regional administrations have the authority to force their constituent Districts to get together and work out what is required.

Administrative and organizational barriers
A new and important problem now looming up on the horizon for many mental hospitals in the United Kingdom is connected with the unstable nature of the final stages of running down and closure of the hospitals. In the first stages of the whole process, the medical staff are liable to be praised as the numbers fall from the previous unacceptably large numbers to more modest levels. This is illustrated in Fig. 17.1. As the number of long-stay patients falls (accompanied by transfer of some of the acute admission beds to District General Hospital units), it soon becomes apparent that large areas of the institutional building are becoming empty or only partly used. Laundries, canteens, gardening departments and boiler houses all become too big for the diminishing population, yet few economies can be made since the basic fabric of the large buildings must be retained, and kept warm and dry. Many hospitals in the United Kingdom are now at this stage and the psychiatrists working in them now find that they are being criticised for being inefficient instead of being given increased praise and support as they approach a very critical period. In addition, the loss of some or all of the acute beds into nearby District General Hospital units can give rise to severe problems in replacing and recruiting sufficient nursing staff to keep the institution going at all, particularly if it is in an isolated rural location.

It seems likely that there will soon emerge in the United Kingdom another form of resistance to the final closure of mental hospitals, this time, perhaps surprisingly, from the psychiatrists themselves, even though they have up to now worked willingly towards run-down and closure. This resistance originates from the somewhat belated recognition that there is much more in a large mental hospital

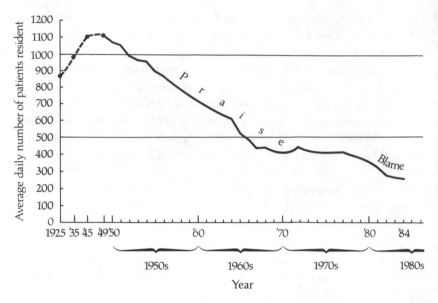

Fig. 17.1. Mapperley Hospital, Nottingham (main building). Average daily number of patients resident, 1925–1984.

than just the acute and the long-stay patients. To use Mapperley Hospital as an example, it contains in addition to acute and long-stay patients, a Postgraduate Psychiatric Training headquarters with secretarial offices, a library, and lecture room facilities. There is also a Medical Records Department which serves all the parts of the psychiatric services, wherever they happen to be in the town. There is a set of offices for the central administration of the psychiatric services of the whole town, plus smaller groups of offices for the heads of nursing, psychiatric social work and clinical psychology. Clustered around the large old buildings are smaller modern units which house the academic department of psychiatry, the drugs and alcohol dependence unit, the psychotherapy unit, the child and adolescent services, and a separate psychiatric outpatient department. Part of the rehabilitation service is also based in the hospital, and there is a day industrial therapy unit, as well as extensive occupational therapy workshops. It was realized, as plans were made for the relocation of some of these services in smaller units at some distance from the present hospital, that there is a considerable risk of destroying the coherence and identity of the psychiatric professions if the hospital is simply closed and the site sold, (which is what the local National Health Service administration has very much in mind). It is difficult to imagine how it would be possible to run an efficient psychiatric service with each of the components listed above dotted around the town in small domestic-scale premises. Without the central base, in this case the mental hospital, the staff would rarely meet.

The need for the administrative and professional base provided by the old institution is highlighted by the paradoxical relationship between changes in numbers of patients and professional staff. For instance, since the founding of the University Department of Psychiatry at Mapperley Hospital in 1971, the number of patients staying overnight in the hospital has roughly halved, but the number of doctors and nurses has roughly doubled. We also now have many more social workers, psychologists and occupational therapists. In other words, we have many more and many different types of professional staff looking after far fewer patients, if only inpatients are taken into account. The total number of new psychiatric referrals to the service has stayed at about the same level over these years, so an interested politician or economist might well ask what we are all doing now. The first part of the reply is that many more patients are seen in outpatient clinics, domiciliary visits and off-site liaison services than in previous years. The second part of the reply is that the old institutions were a very cheap and efficient way of caring for large numbers of psychiatric patients. They can remain so, but only at the cost of continuing to accept the standards of psychiatric care and social ethics of previous generations.

Viewed in this way, it is clear that the running down and the eventual closure of the large psychiatric institutions is a far more complicated process than originally anticipated, with consequences that go far beyond the comparatively simple requirements of the short-stay and the long-stay patients. There are considerable dangers for the identity and cohesion of mental health care professions whose members now need to be alert and prepared to protect themselves and their own interests; indirectly they will also be protecting the interests of the patients who rely upon the network of services. The service administration and the other medical and surgical disciplines show only indifference to this problem up to now and perhaps some of the members even welcome the prospect of the dissolution of what they regard as unnecessary psychiatric empires.

As a footnote to this somewhat alarming message it is worth noting that one rational solution is to develop what might be called a 'District Psychiatric Centre'. This is very definitely not a large hospital but is a geographically close group of small, purpose-designed units, each fulfilling one of the various functions listed above. This concept would allow the professionals concerned to be near enough to each other to survive as a multidisciplinary group, and also in their own right as individual disciplines; with small, modern and well-spaced buildings on a small campus the problems of an institution could be avoided. It may well often turn out that a part of the old mental hospital site will be the obvious place for such a development, so long as the old institutional building itself is demolished. The main disadvantage of this rational approach is its cost, but it is up to psychiatry and related professions to fight hard enough to get the resources needed; there is little doubt that our patients and our professions have been sadly neglected over the last 50 years or so.

Obstacles to multidisciplinary team-work

Although there are numerous reports in the literature of specific instances of multidisciplinary teams being formed sporadically as a result of individual initiatives at different times and places, it seems likely that recently there has been a more general ground-swell of development in the United Kingdom of multidisciplinary team work as a result of a series of changes in the professions concerned – principally an increase in the number and type of professions that are now working in mental health services. There has also been a steady rise in the standards of basic and professional education and training of social workers, nurses and occupational therapists, and to a lesser extent, an improvement in the training of psychiatrists and psychologists. Mental hospitals and psychiatric units are no longer run by self-trained psychiatrists, supported by ''attendants' and part-time voluntary 'lady almoners'. We now have psychiatrists who have postgraduate qualifications following accredited training courses and examinations, we have social workers with degrees and diplomas, and we have nurses with much higher standards of background education, organized nurse training courses, and occasionally university degrees. However, simple proliferation of numbers of staff and types of training does not necessarily bring cooperation and team work, so it is useful to discuss here different ways of interdisciplinary working.

Multidisciplinary practice

Working relationships between the professions have evolved gradually, and various degrees of what is best called 'multidisciplinary practice' have been in existence for twenty years or more; I have personally experienced several different stages of this. For instance, when I was a psychiatric registrar (resident) at the Maudsley Hospital in the late 1950s, experienced members of all the above disciplines were attached to the consultant psychiatrists, and contributed to the assessment, treatment, and management of the patients. But they did not do this as a team in any real sense. It was common practice in those days for the consultant and the junior medical staff to sit in the side room of the ward and discuss in great detail the history of the patient, followed by an interview with the patient. During various stages of these assessments and discussions the ward sister, the occupational therapist, a social worker and a clinical psychologist attached to the consultant would join the group for varying but usually quite short periods of time, to contribute information and opinions. However, the final decisions would be made by the consultant, and these decisions would then be conveyed to those who needed to know them by either the ward sister or the junior doctor. The junior doctor was automatically assumed to be the main agent or key therapist for all the patients, except for specific opinions, assessments, or tasks allocated by the consultant to the social worker and the clinical psychologist. Decisions were rarely made outside the ward rounds, and both the junior doctor and the nursing staff were accustomed to waiting until the next ward round to have their suggestions approved by the consultant. This is certainly multidisciplinary practice from the patient's point of view, but it is not real teamwork from the point of view of the professionals.

The fully developed multi-disciplinary team

Personal clinical experience in a variety of general psychiatric units, together with an opportunity to review a number of psychiatric emergency and crisis intervention services (Cooper, 1979; Katschnig, Cooper & Konieczna, 1990) leads to the suggestion that it is now possible to identify a number of criteria by which a more fully developed style of interdisciplinary work can be recognized; the participants can properly be called a team. The criteria are as follows:–

1. The team is composed of at least three separate disciplines (nearly always containing psychiatry and psychiatric nursing, plus variable numbers of social workers, clinical psychologists and occupational therapists). The members of the team are identified as individuals, and are constant members of the team rather than occasionally attending to represent their department or discipline.

2. All the members of the team must openly acknowledge that they are members, and must know the individual identity of all the other members. (This may sound curious, but it is justified later.)

3. This identified team holds regular meetings to discuss both (a) general team policies, and (b) specific treatments and management programs for individual patients and families.

4. It is agreed by all members of the team that some degree of blurring of roles and sharing of responsibility is useful, as far as the different training, experience, and legal and ethical responsibilities of individual team members allow.

5. The team has agreed policies which make it possible always to identify (a) a team leader, when required (particularly at times of emergency and crisis), (b) a key worker for each patient. The role of key-worker is not restricted to the members of any one profession.

6. It is agreed that most of the contacts with the patient and family will be made by the key-worker, who will be expected to make a variety of day-to-day decisions without necessarily referring these first to other and more professionally senior members of the team. The number and type

of these day-to-day decisions will depend upon the experience and qualifications of the key-worker. Major decisions (such as time of admission or discharge) will always be discussed with the team.

This more fully developed style of multidisciplinary team work is well known and quite well publicized by enthusiasts, but, although it is spreading, it is probably still not very common in the United Kingdom. Almost everybody in psychiatry nowadays claims to work in a multidisciplinary team style, but a closer examination of what actually happens in many units usually demonstrates that they are following some variety or other of the older style of multidisciplinary practice. The commonest anomaly found is that the consultant psychiatrist claims to be working by means of a multidisciplinary team, and the alleged members of this team deny any knowledge of it. According to descriptions of various psychiatric services in both the United States and the United Kingdom, it seems clear that the most extreme varieties of this multidisciplinary style of work (extreme in the sense of the psychiatrist devolving most, if not all, of his traditional responsibilities to the members of other disciplines) have developed in the two wings of the psychiatric services (also extreme from the point of view of urgency of decisions and speed of turnover of patients). These are, first, crisis intervention and emergency psychiatric units, which have a comparatively large turnover of short-stay patients needing many and urgent decisions, and second, rehabilitation units and day centres, where patients move through the service comparatively slowly and decisions are rarely urgent. The common element shared by these two apparently very different wings of the psychiatric services is that most of the decisions being made are to do with social and psychological problems and management issues not requiring detailed medical or psychiatric knowledge. These are appropriate to be shared or dealt with completely by nonmedical members of the team.

Who should be the leader of the team?
There is no simple answer, since such teams may work in different settings with different responsibilities. But for teams working in a clearly medical framework, such as a psychiatric hospital or psychiatric unit in a general hospital, there is surely only one possible answer – the leader should be a psychiatrist. In contrast, teams in different settings, such as extramural day-centres, rehabilitations units, crisis units or social service departments may well have leaders from the nonmedical disciplines. This distinction is based upon the legal and ethical responsibilities possessed by the medical profession that are imposed upon it by society, together with responsibilities for medication and investigations. The consequences of having a medical leader for an individual team cannot be spelled out in detail, because there are many ways of being a leader most of which depend upon the personalities involved in the team. Long discussions are possible about types and

styles of leadership, but it is only necessary to say here that the sort of leader being implied is not a dominant or domineering role. In most of the day-to-day discussions, there may well be no obvious team leader; the discussion of each problem or patient gets a different and informal mediator or chairman in turn, as a natural development. The agreed leader emerges as such only when disagreements cannot be resolved easily, or when basic policies or strategies are in danger of being ignored or need developing afresh.

Systematic studies which show that the multidisciplinary team style of work is 'better' than its predecessors, judged on measures such as speed or completeness of recovery, cost, safety, and rate of turnover of patients, are not available. Indeed, such studies would be very difficult, if not impossible to carry out in practice. There is simply a general assumption that the multidisciplinary method is preferable; it is certainly spreading, in spite of this lack of any systematic evidence in its favour. Job satisfaction on the part of the team members who are not psychiatrists is probably one of the major influences in this increasing popularity.

Problems between disciplines; authority, training and responsibility
What professional influences help or hinder the development of the spread of this multidisciplinary team work between disciplines? A whole complex of problems can easily be identified here concerned with issues such as the development and identity of the professions of psychology and social work, and their wish to break away from the traditional authority exercised over them by psychiatrists. These feelings are partly the natural consequences of the development of techniques and expertise unique to the newer professions. There is also some resentment about the past, remembering the way in which psychiatrists were sometimes accustomed to giving instructions to psychologists and social workers, even though they had little understanding of what the members of these professions could do.

Disagreements still exist about who has authority over whom in dealing with patients, and to what extent the different professions are responsible for different aspects of the patients. It is therefore worthwhile to consider here in some detail the differences in training of the different professions, since this will presumably lead to a clarification of the responsibilities appropriate to the members of the different professions. The following section summarizes briefly the different backgrounds and qualifications of the professions concerned. Fig. 17.2 illustrates the length and nature of the training of general practitioners, psychiatrists, clinical psychologists, psychiatric nurses, social workers and occupational therapists. Qualifications for entry to the different professional courses vary somewhat in European countries, but the generalizations discussed here are based primarily upon those in the United Kingdom and the United States. There are, of course, always a few exceptional individuals with double qualifications or obvious

	General practitioner	Psychiatrist	Clinical psychologist	Social worker	Psychiatric nurse	Occupational therapist
Entry qualifications	very high	very high	high	high	lowest	moderately high
Length to university graduation or first degree	5 or 6 years	5 or 6 years	3 years	3 years	3 years	3 years
Length of postgraduate course	1+3 years	1+3+3 years	3 years	3 years	2 years	3 years
Total time to responsibility	9 or 10 years	12–13 years	6 years	6 years	5 years	6 years
Variety of topics in training:						
Physical	+++	++	-	-	+	++
Psychological	+	++	+++	+	+	++
Social	+	++	++	+++	++	-
Psychiatric	+	+++	+	+	+	+

Fig. 17.2. Comparison of length and variety of training for members of psychiatric multidisciplinary teams (all figures are approximate).

academic underachievement in every discipline, but it is necessary here to consider the 'average' or 'expected' standards and abilities.

Competition is usually keenest for entry to medical schools. The academic achievement required for a place in a medical school tends to be higher than for a place on a psychology degree course or diploma. Occupational therapy requirements are somewhat lower than these two, and entry standards for nursing training come last on the list. (Differences between nurses in the United States and the United Kingdom need further discussion.)

The extent of responsibility for patients is an important point which is often neglected. The doctors have an overall legal and ethical responsibility for what happens to patients, and this cannot be avoided. In the British National Health Service this is a 24 hours a day commitment, and there is always a doctor on duty representing this responsibility. The same applies to the nurses, in terms of responsibility for the physical welfare of the patients; again there is cover for the 24 hours by means of shifts and teams. The other professions do not have this responsibility and therefore are not troubled by night or week-end duties (with the recent exception of Social Workers in the United Kingdom.) This reflects the 'partial' nature of what they do with the patients in the day-time – the psychologist and the social workers are not responsible for the physical state or medication of the patient, and the occupational therapist is not responsible for those parts of the patient's day that are outside a defined program of activities.

In contrast, the psychiatrist or general practitioner are the only ones whose training enables them to survey, from time to time, *all* aspects of the patient and his problems – the lengthy medical and psychiatric training has included aspects of the main elements of the training courses of all the other disciplines, at one stage or another. This is not to pretend that the psychiatrist is automatically as competent in everything as members of the other professions, but he should have a working knowledge and appreciation of what they can do. Furthermore, he should have this to a greater extent than they can be expected to know about his own specific medical and psychiatric responsibilities. In particular, the other professions know little about the potentially dangerous areas to do with physical illness, medication, physical investigations and physical treatments. These differing degrees of completeness of responsibility, hours of duty, and understanding of the activities of others, lie behind the uneasiness of many doctors when faced with demands for equality between the professions in a multidisciplinary team.

The gradient of danger
In discussing these different responsibilities in different disciplines of the medical profession, it is possible to see a 'gradient of danger' which is related to the extent to which responsibility and equality are demanded by other professions. When the medical and surgical disciplines deal with dangerous and acute illness, delegation

of responsibility or blurring of roles are hardly mentioned. The dangers of delegation diminish for the patient as one moves from considering surgical or medical teams towards psychiatric ones. Moving from acute general psychiatric work to work with long-stay patients continues the same process, and in working with highly selected crisis patients, (see also Katschnig Chap. 7), the medical dangers may perhaps be least. It is therefore not surprising that it is in this type of work that the demands for sharing of responsibility are most obvious and most appropriate.

As the discussion passes down this gradient of danger, we can see that differences between the setting and purpose of the medical teams will impose different structures and methods of work. A medical anthropologist or medical sociologist would predict that the presence of dangerous situations would necessitate the emergence of structure, status, and clear lines of responsibility; set rules will exist and a certain number of rituals should be fairly obvious, since they have important reassuring functions. In the less acute and often more specialized teams (e.g. rehabilitation day hospitals and day centres) where there are fewer urgent and dangerous problems one would expect a less obvious structure, fewer needs for status, and less clear lines of decision-making; rituals should be less obvious.

Reciprocal understanding between disciplines

There appears to be a considerable ignorance of the professions about the training and knowledge of each other. This can be seen in a particularly clear manner when one examines the curricula of nurse training courses, or social work diplomas. It is often found that nurses are teaching psychiatry to nurses, and psychologists are teaching psychiatry to psychologists, rather than these disciplines enrolling psychiatric teachers to teach psychiatry. (It is sometimes easy to discover a policy of positive avoidance of using teachers from their parent disciplines.) On the whole, in most psychiatric training courses, psychologists teach psychology to the psychiatrists, but it is possible to find psychologists who are reluctant to teach psychiatrists. Sadly, it is very unusual to find anybody teaching anything about nursing to psychiatrists (or to any other type of doctor).

This lack of reciprocal teaching contacts is presumably one of the reasons for the ignorance of most of the members of the team about exactly what it is that the other members from different disciplines have been trained to do. This has already been mentioned between the disciplines as a whole, but it is also appropriate to bring it in at the individual level, since this is where it often becomes manifest. In the United Kingdom few members of the nonmedical disciplines in the team have very much idea of the sequence of referral and 'filtration' through which a patient passes before he comes to see a psychiatrist. (Goldberg & Huxley, 1980). In the United Kingdom and in some European countries there is a well-developed primary care system interposed between the general public and the specialists. In the United States, this is far more patchy, but the absence of a filtration or gatekeeper system will serve to increase rather than diminish the anxieties of the psychiatrist in the team about the possible consequences of delegation of responsibility. It is the responsibility of the general practitioner in the primary care service to check that the physical state of the patient is normal or that any abnormalities have been dealt with, before referring the patient to a general psychiatrist.

The general psychiatrist, too, also has in mind the possibility of accompanying or underlying physical illness when taking even a clearly psychiatric history, and he may well check the patient's physical state again. Patients are also often referred to a psychiatrist during a period of changing symptoms, and the clinical picture and the associated problems may be very different by the time of the psychiatric consultation a week or two later. Physical conditions previously masked may emerge, and more serious psychiatric illnesses such as schizophrenia or sever depression may gradually develop. The general psychiatrist is trained to bear these things in mind, and always should keep his eyes and ears open for unpleasant physical possibilities. Nurses are also trained to remember this aspect of psychiatric care, but psychologists and social workers are often unaware or only partly aware of these dangers; they are also often unaware of the sequence of referral and 'filtration'. They often do not realize that patients seen by multidisciplinary psychiatric teams are highly selected, and may not appreciate why the omission of any of these selection and checking processes make a general psychiatrist feel uneasy.

A closely related problem is that psychologists and social workers are often very surprised to witness the wide variety of problems, decisions and types of patients faced by a general psychiatrist when he is acting as an important part of the selection and filtration process during the course of a busy general psychiatric outpatient clinic. For instance, a mixed bag of five or six patients, often with family members also to be seen, may set problems ranging from the effects of injectable phenothiazines on the sex life of a young man with chronic schizophrenia, to demands for facial plastic surgery from a young woman of apparently normal appearance. I have found that by getting psychologists and social workers to sit in with me during one or two of these general clinics produces a reaction of surprise, and they admit readily they had had no previous idea of the variety of problems presented to a general psychiatrist. It is very important that the other disciplines should be aware of the 'gradient of danger' that psychiatrists and general practitioners have been trained to keep in mind. Another long debate is possible about how justified is this cautious medical attitude, and to what extent is it maintained by a fear of litigation (or, in private practice, by hope of profit).

Conceptual models of ill health

Psychiatrists are often puzzled when social workers and psychologists accuse them of being preoccupied by or limited to 'the medical model' when thinking about their patients. It is worthwhile therefore to mention briefly the conceptual models of ill health that seem to guide the thinking and reactions of the various professions during both training and daily clinical work. 'Disease' models, 'medical' models, and models of social and cognitive learning are the concepts concerned.

Social workers naturally learn about social models, and psychologists tend to concentrate upon models based upon learning theory and cognitive processes. They are all too fond of assuming that all doctors automatically think only in terms of physical disease and physical processes, but in doing so they make a serious mistake. As we have seen, because of the 'gradient of danger' the doctors are trained to think first of possible physical diseases as an explanation of what the patients present, but they are also trained to move on to other models if no physical diseases are found. This is particularly so for psychiatrists. Nowadays, all psychiatric training courses contain extensive sections on social psychology and sometimes even medical anthropology; illness behaviour and the sick role are discussed, and the relevance of viewing the same patient in different ways is emphasized. In other words, the 'medical' model that is so beloved of the nonmedical disciplines is a misnomer. The model used by doctors should be a sequence of several models in order of clinical importance and danger. The first is the physical or disease model, and discussion then moves to the psychological and the social models, all being used in succession with respect to one patient and his family.

Intramedical problems

Within the psychiatric discipline of the medical profession, there is at the moment a generation gap in terms of education and in terms of appreciation of psychosocial issues. It is probably just about at its peak now and should disappear over the next five to ten years. Senior psychiatrists in practice at the moment (in the last five years or so of their career) are from the generation who had no behavioural sciences training in their undergraduate course, little supervised study during their psychiatric training and often had to teach themselves clinical psychiatry under very difficult conditions in large mental hospitals. They did this while caring for large numbers of patients, with little or no support from other disciplines. They are now faced with a generation of junior doctors who have gone through extensive behaviour sciences courses in their medical schools, who have had teaching on patient/doctor communication and interviewing techniques, and are probably in the middle of quite extensive postgraduate psychiatric courses containing elements of psychology, sociology and related subjects. These senior consultants also find themselves in contact with nurses preoccupied with 'the nursing process', keen and willing to take decisions and responsibility upon their newly qualified shoulders. However broad minded these senior consultants may try to be, it must be extremely difficult for them to adjust to the new generation of workers and to the multidisciplinary team approach. Nevertheless, they still have a great deal of authority and influence in their clinical practice, particularly if they remain within the large mental hospitals. This is probably a contributing influence to the rather slow development and spread of neighbourhood psychiatry and multidisciplinary team work in many parts of the United Kingdom. Perhaps the present patchy distribution will gradually even out over the next few years, simply as a result of the passage of time.

Possible remedies for the future

What can be done to diminish these problems and barriers that have been identified? With regard to the problems that came under the general heading of the development of the strategies of mental health care, such as the move out of the mental hospitals and the development of neighbourhood psychiatry, perhaps attention could be given to the roles of the different professionals in both the long-term and the short-term planning process.

It is easy to recommend joint planning at the higher levels, that is, between government departments, and between the District Health Authorities of the National Health Service and the local Social Services Committees. Unfortunately, we have in the United Kingdom far too many examples of non-cooperation at these levels to be optimistic about the effect of this simple and rational advice. For instance, even in the presence of officially labelled 'Joint Planning Committees' between District Health Authorities and the local Social Services Committee, there is often little to see as a result. This may be because these two types of organizations are very different sorts of animals. A District Health Authority is comparatively nonpolitical, whereas a Social Services Committee is clearly dominated by one of the local political parties but the dominance may swing the other way after the next local political election. I have had experience of being one of the psychiatric members of such a Joint Planning Team, which was presented with detailed and comprehensive two and five-year psychiatric plans. The Social Service representatives (otherwise quite reasonable individuals) could only apologize for the absence of equivalent plans with which the psychiatric plans could be co-ordinated. It was the policy of the Social Services Committee of that time *not* to have plans that went more than about six months into the future. Something was achieved by personal contact on a small scale, but there was much frustration all round. This illustrates the impotence of professional organisations when faced with political or administrative bodies who control the money in the long term.

It is often not appreciated, at least in the United Kingdom, that the medical profession has had very little say in the major decisions about the design of the health services. For instance, nobody knows who provided the detailed advice upon which 'Better Services for the Mentally Ill' was based: this is the 'blueprint' published in 1975, upon which government policy has since been based. (HMSO 1975). Similarly, mental hospitals were not built at the suggestion of psychiatrists, and psychiatrists have not been responsible as a profession for planning their run-down and closure. There is, in fact, a tripartite report in existence, published jointly by the British Medical Association, the Royal College of Psychiatrists and the Society of Medical Officers of Health, which expresses doubts and reservations about some of the basic policies of the British Government for the development of mental health services. The report is in favour of the general trend out of the large hospitals into other types of facility, but urges caution rather than haste (The Tripartite Committee, 1972). Their warnings are now being shown to have had substance.

With regard to the improvement in reciprocal understanding between the professions, it is easy to suggest that each discipline should teach the students of other disciplines about its own subject. If not, then the organizers of the course should be required to explain why their students should hear about their future professional colleagues only at second hand. In addition, part of the regular activities of a multidisciplinary team should be occasional but regular explanatory sessions in which each discipline would explain exactly what they think they can do better than, or as well as, the other members of the team.

It is probably at the local and individual level that most can be done to achieve smooth progress in developing and promulgating new developments. Small groups of individuals in the different disciplines who can tolerate or even welcome the different viewpoints of each other can often achieve a surprising amount even with scanty resources. It is no use merely to wait to be given both plans and money – they rarely come together, and when they do it is all too easy to waste some of the money by going too quickly. Small pilot or trial schemes, organized by key individuals and groups, can set the scene and demonstrate how advances in services can be made; if they are notably successful, they may generate their own support and spread simply by example. Failing this, a small-scale development can survive until more resources come along, keeping going largely on staff satisfaction and internal stability. It takes many years for a new idea or attitude to permeate the medical profession, perhaps even a generation. For instance, in the United Kingdom the practice of consultant psychiatrists spending some of their time on primary care premises (perhaps only an hour or so per week) has been around for 20 years. But in the last five years or so it has begun to spread rapidly and it is now a very significant factor in working relationships between the two parts of the medical profession. A survey in 1984 showed that 25 % of psychiatrists were involved in primary care visiting, and this is probably an underestimate (Strathdee & Williams, 1986).

As members of a profession who are supposed to have some insight into the behaviour of both individuals and groups, psychiatrists must be wary of large scale changes suddenly imposed from the outside; it is better to concentrate upon the more gradual diffusion of practices based upon successful co-operation between individuals and small groups who have discovered how to trust and learn from each other.

Acknowledgements

I am most grateful to Mr Stanley Woollerton, Medical Records Officer, Mapperley Hospital, for the information from which Figure 17.1 is constructed.

References

Cooper, J. E. (1979). *Crisis Admission Units and Emergency Psychiatric Services* Public Health in Europe Series: No 11 W.H.O. Copenhagen.

Goldberg, D. & Huxley, P. (1980). *Mental Illness in the Community: the pathway to psychiatric care.* Tavistock Publications: London and New York.

HMSO (1975). *Better Services For the Mentally Ill.* Reprinted 1980. HMSO.

The Tripartite Committee (1972). *The Mental Health Service after Unification:* Royal College of Psychiatrists, Society of Medical Officers of Health, and British Medical Association: Publ.: Underhill (Plymouth) for BMA.

Katschnig, H., Cooper, J. E. & Konieczna, T. (1990). Emergency psychiatry and crisis intervention services in Europe. In *Community Psychiatry* (Bennett, & Freeman, eds), Churchill Livingstone: London (in press).

Strathdee, G. & Williams, P. (1986). Patterns of Collaboration. *In Mental Illness in Primary Care Settings* (Shepherd, M., Wilkinson, G. & Williams, P. eds), Tavistock Publications: New York and London.

Commentary on Chapter 17

Mary Ann Test and Isaac M. Marks

Professional issues and obstacles are enormously important but often neglected. They include larger-scale economic and organizational factors. The type of practice that professionals choose to spend their time on is crucial to the success and dissemination of innovative programs. Staff represent a tremendous resource. In all disciplines there are many competent staff capable of doing far more than they are given credit or responsibility for. Most want high job satisfaction and can gain this by doing what is effective. Currently in the United States large numbers of mental health staff service the least needy, the worried well. And even those serving the most needy are often implementing ineffective treatment rather than today's more helpful innovations. How can this powerful and necessary resource be harnessed?

John Cooper mentioned several important obstacles. One not discussed is how to attract professional staff to work in public psychiatry with chronic psychotic people in an innovative way as part of an interdisciplinary community team. In the United States most psychiatrists, psychologists and social workers avoid working with such clients, preferring to do private practice psychodynamic psychotherapy on their own. In social work, students who choose mental health want to be psychotherapists. Training programs reflect that interest. There are only four training programs in the United States for social workers to work with the chronic mentally ill.

There are many reasons for this drift in the United States toward private practice psychotherapy, away from work with chronic psychotic patients. Care for them carries low salaries and low status. In contrast, the public is fascinated with psychodynamic theory and therapy, and professionals perceive greater gratification from such therapy, which seems to give greater intimacy with clients, and

254

purportedly 'cures' or 'heals' rather than merely rehabilitating and maintaining the function of clients. 'Doing therapy' seems to afford greater work challenges than the hustling for jobs and living situations of chronic psychotic people who are thought to be unattractive. Few good, satisfied professional models are available. Private practice seems to give greater autonomy without a wrestle with interdisciplinary issues or being 'number two' in a staff hierarchy.

In the United Kingdom many of these issues are less salient than in the United States. There are fewer differential fiscal incentives to work with the worried well rather than with chronic psychosis. Public psychiatry has higher status and recognition in the United Kingdom, and rehabilitation approaches are more accepted.

The area needs to be marketed differently to attract professionals into the field. Higher pay is needed for the work, with all disciplines lobbying for it together. Professionals need to be trained and encouraged to implement what works rather than to do inappropriate psychotherapy for chronic psychosis. They need to get into the interdisciplinary issues that John Cooper discussed.

Who should do this work? One option is to continue the present system of having several professionals working in multidiciplinary teams, but to teach them to work together more smoothly. Alternatively, a new type of care provider for chronic psychosis could be trained, but such a group would probably end up having low status and losing public attention. Other disciplines would be able to dump the problem onto the new providers, get off the hook, and lose interest. They would stop advocating for chronic psychotic people or for better pay of the new providers, who would end up with the same low status and low pay fate as 'social casework', which no one wants to do.

How can people be attracted into the field? There are no easy answers. It needs the best minds and staff from all disciplines. More model programs staffed by interdisciplinary teams are required. People need to be educated into realizing that work with chronic psychosis needs much greater biopsychosocial skills than doing psychotherapy with more motivated people, and is not just a question of babysitting and plugging clients into existing resources. Working with the most difficult patients demands the greater skills in psychiatry, as in other fields like open heart surgery. It requires knowledge of symptoms and their complex interaction with environmental factors and stresses. It needs dealing with individual patients and with public attitudes and resistance. Gaining the trust of a paranoid patient and of a landlord in whose dwelling that patients wants to live is far harder than doing therapy with a motivated college student.

A different training is required that is truly interdisciplinary, encouraging role expansions rather than turf guarding and argument over who is responsible. All disciplines need to be prepared, trained and encouraged to take more responsibility for the difficult work involved. The more that staff know about biological, psychological and sociological processes relevant to chronic psychosis, the more effective they will be in preventing relapse and crisis and in enabling growth.

There are complex power issues. Physicians' attitude that they are 'responsible' can be insulting to other professionals, who should be trained to take more responsibility. The issue may be relevant to aspects of women's liberation, since most physicians are men and most other staff are women. Men can feel relieved when women take more responsibility for themselves.

How can truly interdisciplinary training programs be developed? Trainees from different disciplines need to spend training time together as a team. In the team they can learn to like and respect each other and to teach one another what they know. They should become as interchangeable as possible – when alone on the street with a psychotic patient they need to know what to do with him/her, the community and the family. Who the team leader should be should depend on competence, and the leader need not necessarily be a doctor. Such interdisciplinary training can be stimulating and attractive to staff. A few model training programs of this kind do exist and they work; they need to get more widely known and their methods should become part of the curricula of professional schools. Dissemination doesn't just happen, but has to be deliberately developed. More such interdisciplinary programs have been set up through Robert Wood Johnson Foundation grants.

In conclusion, while the above options should sound ideal, they are supported by the market now. Concerns about containing health care costs support the role expansion and training of each discipline to become as responsible as possible. In the area of professional roles and training the things that make sense therapeutically can also be the things that make sense economically.

18

Implementation and overview

Robert A. Scott & Isaac M. Marks

This international multidisciplinary volume has highlighted both unity and diversity in innovations in mental health care delivery. Worldwide, there are pressures towards cost constraint, value for money, and community care. Also usual is neglect of ways to expand the roles of care providers and self-help even when these give demonstrably good value for money. It has been shown that nurse practitioners like nurse therapists in the United Kingdom obtain good clinical outcomes and lower resource consumption by patients despite shorter training than physicians or psychologists, yet such nurse therapists are still scarce 17 years after they began. Self-help by self-exposure therapy can be effective for phobic and obsessive-compulsive disorders, yet its take-up is slow.

A ubiquitous problem is that of countries formulating and thrusting policy on a country before adequate research has shown what is needed, what policy would best meet that need, and how to evaluate its implementation. Conversely, when good innovative investigations indicate what works well the message is slow to be acted on – useful developments spread sluggishly through mental health care systems. Attitudes and the policies that express them are shaped by wider social forces at least as much as by sound research. And what research is done reflects those forces.

A constant fact of life is that, however clear patient needs might be and knowledge of how to satisfy them, translating that into practice depends on all the vagaries of the political process. Implementation of a hard-won mental health care Act was halted as soon as President Carter was succeeded by President Reagan, the care of subnormality was boosted when President Kennedy's sister happened to be subnormal, abortion in France was liberalized by a woman Health Minister using mistaken statistics. For innovators to succeed it is not enough to do sound scientific research and publicize it. They also have to try to create the 'political will' for change by assiduously cultivating the right contacts and seizing opportunities when they can, knowing that they will still often be blown off course by contrary political winds.

Also omnipresent is the danger that concentrating on innovation may lose lessions from antiquity and waste resources by constantly re-inventing the wheel. Community care is now new; it could benefit from a historical perspective of its many forms over the centuries. 'Deinstitutionalization' as an idea developed years after the trend to discharge patients out of mental hospitals began after World War II, before phenothiazines came in. There seems agreement that community care does not work unless it integrates the various asylum functions outside hospital previously provided by mental hospitals; these include aid with crises, with daily, social and recreational activities, with housing, employment, finance and budgeting, and with medical and mental health care. This need to integrate all asylum functions in the community is recognized in the Robert Wood Johnson Foundation nine-cities initiatives.

The diversity of problems was sharpened by contrasting the decentralized United States political system with the more centralized one in the United Kingdom. Yet even the United Kingdom system conceals great differences within its various parts; the move towards community care has been faster in England than in Scotland. Japan and South Korea have build many new mental hospitals at a time other countries have dismantled them. European countries differ greatly in their patterns of mental health care provision, proportions of different care providers, psychiatric beds, and organization of emergency psychiatric care. There are fascinating opportunities for comparative research across countries that would deepen our understanding of the factors shaping mental care delivery.

More particular differences also operate. United States hospitals are not encouraged to have sheltered workshops; instead, patients learn crisis coping skills that have to be maintained at their normal worksite. What works in some ethnic groups may not in others. A standard treatment for sexual dysfunction in the United States might not be tolerated in Saudi Arabia, so English texts may have to be modified when translated into Arabic.

Although there will always be formidable impediments to the implementation of useful innovations, careful attention to them could quicken the pace of their evolution and dissemination in mental health care delivery.

Index

Author index

Abel Smith, B.   132
Ackerman, S. R.   152
Aiken, L. H.   226, 229, 230, 231
Airing, C. D.   23
Alkire, A. A.   37
Allen, C.   210, 211, 212, 215, 217
Allness, D. J.   11
Amies, P. L.   74
Anderson, E. M.   37
Andrews, G.   74, 75
Ashcroft, G. W.   73
Ashurst, P. M.   75
Atay, J. E.   220, 225, 227
Atkinson, A. B.   127
Austin, A.   74

Backer, T. E.   54
Baling, M.   72
Balter, M. B.   74
Barrett, S. A.   224
Bassuk, E. L.   91, 104
Bedi, H.   19
Beecham, J.   210, 211, 212, 213, 215
Beigel, A.   33
Beitman, B.   64
Bell, R.   152
Belsey, E.   65, 71
Bendix, T.   75
Berkowitz, R.   37
Birk, A. W.   104

Birley, J. L. T.   22
Bishop, S.   74
Blackburn, I. M.   74
Bland, M.   78
Blashki, T. G.   73
Blazer, D. G.   61, 62
Bodison, D.   224
Bosanquet, B.   123
Boyd, L. J.   37
Boyer, C. A.   226, 228
Brandon, S.   25
Braun, P.   11
Breemer ter Stege, C.   158
Bridges, K. W.   26, 28, 63, 65
Briggs, J.   42
Brodaty, H.   74, 75
Brodie, 64
Brown, G. W.   22, 23, 24
Brown, P.   22, 23, 24
Budson, R. D.   23
Buglass, D.   22
Burchell, A.   70, 71, 76, 209
Burke, J. D. Jnr   73
Burns, T. P.   76
Burt, R.   152, 153
Burton, R. H.   63, 72
Byrne, P. S.   76

Cambridge, P.   210, 211, 212, 215, 217
Caroli, F.   91

259

Subject index